Intermittent Fasting

Unlocking the 16:8 Diet to Burn Fat and Activate Autophagy While Still Enjoying Delicious Meals and a Comprehensive IF Guide for Woman Over 50

Contents

Part 1: Intermittent Fasting 16/8

The Effective Weight Loss Guide for Women and Men Wanting to Fast, Burn Fat, and Activate Autophagy While Still Enjoying Delicious Meals

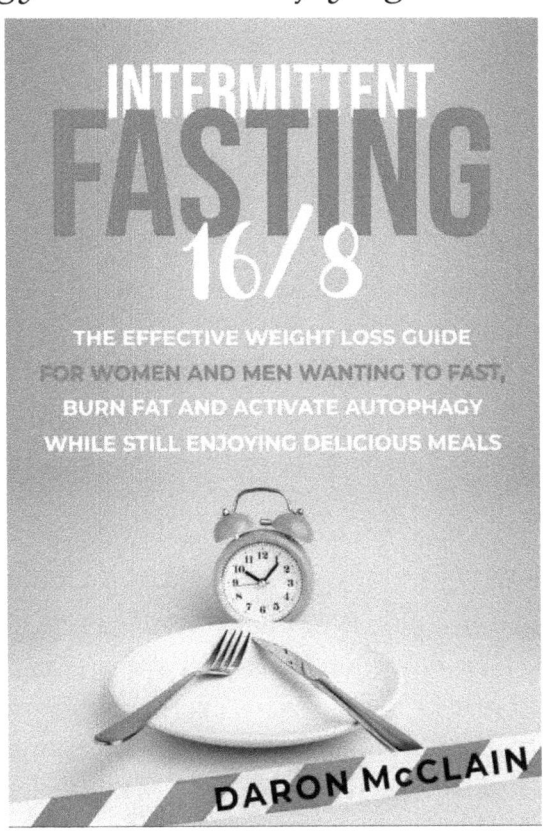

Introduction

Our modern lifestyle is all about convenience and comfort. These two factors also influence what foods we consume and what diets we follow. Most of us don't pay much attention to what we eat or when we eat, which seems to be the primary cause of steadily increasing health problems. The simplest way to remedy all this is by becoming mindful of your diet. Since there are countless diets to choose from, how do you know which one will work best for you? Well, you don't have to look any further because intermittent fasting is for anyone!

The concept of fasting is not new or foreign, and humans have been fasting since time immemorial. Fasting gives your body a much-needed breather to stabilize its internal systems and functions. Intermittent fasting is a protocol that alternates between periods of eating and fasting. It is a great, simple way to optimize your overall health and wellbeing. From weight loss and maintenance to improving heart health, energy levels, and metabolism, there is a lot to gain from it.

You can do all this while enjoying delicious meals. Yes, you read that right! Dieting is no longer synonymous with eating measly portions or starving.

Intermittent fasting is perfectly sustainable in the long run. The 16/8 protocol is one of the most popular forms of intermittent fasting. You essentially fast for sixteen hours daily while the eating window is restricted to eight hours on this diet. During these eight hours, you can consume three healthy, wholesome, and delicious meals. By becoming mindful of your diet, paying attention to the food choices you make, and adding a little exercise to your daily life, you can achieve your weight loss and fitness goals. This is a great way to quickly burn fat by engaging your body's metabolism.

This book will teach you the meaning of intermittent fasting, how it works, and the various benefits it offers. The 16/8 intermittent fasting protocol is quite easy to follow and can be readily adjusted according to your preferences and lifestyle. This book contains plenty of practical tips you can follow to transition to this diet effortlessly. It also contains steps to improve your chances of success and a few common intermittent fasting mistakes you need to avoid. Apart from that, this book also includes a detailed guide of what you can and cannot eat while following this diet, how to break your fast, and what you can consume during the fasting period.

In all aspects of life, motivation is important, and dieting is no different. By following the simple suggestions in this book on staying motivated and tackling fasting setbacks, your chances of success are bound to increase. You will also learn tips to help you add exercise to your daily routine, and gain an understanding of how your metabolism affects your ability to gain or lose weight. All in all, this book will act as your transitional guide toward intermittent fasting.

Lastly, this book includes several 16/8 intermittent fasting recipes and a detailed meal plan to help get you started. All the recipes in this book are super nutritious and incredibly simple to prepare without compromising taste or flavor. You need not worry about counting calories to lose weight. Simply pay attention to *when* you eat—this is the only change you need to make. Forget about spending hours in the kitchen cooking diet-friendly meals. Once you start cooking the suggested recipes in this book, your idea of cooking will change for the better. Following a diet has never been this easy and accessible. Or this fun!

Chapter 1: The Science of Fasting

Most health problems we face nowadays are primarily caused by our modern diets. This is where fasting steps in. As a time-tested ancient tradition, fasting has been a part of human life since time immemorial. Whether for spiritual or medical reasons, fasting is quite a common practice.

One of the biggest misconceptions people have about fasting is that it is synonymous with starvation. Unless you change your mindset about fasting, you cannot make it a part of your daily lifestyle. The difference is that starvation is involuntary and is caused by the absence of food. In contrast, fasting is a deliberate, conscious, and therefore controlled act. You never know where your next meal will come from or when you can eat again with starvation. When voluntarily abstaining from consuming any solid foods, this is known as fasting. Fasting is not only natural but steadily gaining popularity in health and fitness communities worldwide.

History of Fasting

Fasting is an ancient healing tradition practiced by most cultures and religions across the globe. Hippocrates, considered to be the father of modern science, was a staunch proponent of regular fasting. A common treatment he prescribed was fasting and consuming apple cider vinegar on an empty stomach to promote one's health. He believed that eating while sick merely makes the illness fester. Plutarch, an ancient Greek writer and historian, had similar sentiments. He believed that it is best to make fasting a part of your daily life instead of depending on medicine and treatment. Other famous Greek thinkers such as Plato and Aristotle also backed these claims. They all believed fasting could be used as prevention and cure.

This goes to show how ancient Greeks believed medical treatment and options could be inspired by nature. In fact, most animals don't usually eat when they're sick; this is one reason why fasting is labeled as "the physician within your body." It is the basic instinct that makes animals such as cats or dogs effectively anorexic when sick. However, it is not just animals. Even humans experience reduced appetite when they are unwell. Take a moment and think about it: back when you were sick with the flu, you probably realized that eating was the last thing on your mind. Even foods you normally crave suddenly seem unappetizing when you're sick. This is your body's way of inducing an automatic fast to heal itself. The human body is quite intuitive, and it usually knows what it needs to heal and repair itself. Fasting is a part of our human instinct and is deeply embedded into our biological heritage. Sadly, though, most of us ignore these cues and treat our bodies as tireless machines.

Another popular belief about fasting is that it can help improve your cognitive abilities. If you take a moment and think about it, it makes perfect sense. How do you feel after a heavy and greasy meal made up of carbs and sugars? Chances are you feel quite tired and sluggish. You certainly do not feel energetic. Reduction in your energy levels and sluggishness are both associated with the heavy food you consume. Most of your body's blood supply is directed to the digestive system after a heavy meal to digest the food you have just consumed. This, in turn, reduces the blood supply available to other organs, especially the brain. This results in lethargy and drowsiness. You are essentially inducing your body into a state of "food coma" by eating heavy meals. When you start fasting regularly, this process is reversed.

Aside from fasting for health reasons, fasting is also widely considered a spiritual practice. It is commonly practiced in many religions and cultures across the globe. Whether in Hinduism, Islam, Christianity, Judaism, Jainism, or Buddhism, fasting is a sacred practice. It is used as a means for spiritual enlightenment and purification. Several religious scriptures suggest fasting has healing powers. It is also believed to purge your soul of all sins you may have committed. Another popular religious notion holds that fasting helps connect your body, mind, and soul.

During the holy month of Ramadan, Muslims fast from sunrise until sunset. Islamic scriptures suggest fasting twice a week is good for your body and soul. Likewise, Buddhist monks are known for observing strict fasts quite frequently. Even Hindu scripture describes similar notions. So, it is safe to say that fasting is not a modern concept and has managed to stand the test of time.

Understanding the "Fasted" and "Fed" States of the Body

There are several misconceptions about fasting, which we now know are myths. Fasting does not harm your body. To understand how it works, you need to differentiate between the two primary states of the human body: "fasted" and "fed" states. Your body is in either of these states at all times. It cannot be in both states simultaneously.

Humans have evolved and all the amenities, innovations, and technology at our disposal have made our lives rather convenient. Convenience and choice are two characteristics of the modern lifestyle. This is especially true for our diet these days. Walk into any grocery store, and you will see multiple options. When so many snacks and food options are available, constant snacking has become the norm. Most of us are used to snacking on something or other throughout the day. Whenever you eat, your body is in a fed state. In this state, your body primarily focuses on the digestion, absorption, and assimilation of the food you consume.

As you eat, the food is transformed into energy by your body's internal metabolism. All of this energy is not immediately used, and a portion of it is stored for later. This is a part of our evolutionary mechanism to ensure survival. All the energy in reserve is like your body's personal savings account. Your body dips into this reserve only when there is a shortage of food. This extra energy is stored in the form of fat cells. Since there is no upper limit to the number of fat cells that can be created, your body is equipped to accumulate as much fat as it wants to. This process continues for as long as your body is in a fed state.

On the other hand, a fasted state is one where you abstain from eating, either voluntarily or involuntarily. Your body utilizes those fat reserves during the fasted state. When you don't eat, your body has nothing to do other than depend on its energy resources to keep itself going. Most of us are in a fasted state only when we are sleeping. Think of fasting as a simple extension of this period: as long as you eat, you are in a fed state, and when you stop eating, you are in a fasted state.

A primary law of nature is that there needs to be balance. This is embodied through the Chinese philosophy of Yin and Yang, which symbolizes the importance of balance. This balance is crucial in all aspects of your life, which is the root cause of most problems. This applies to your body, too. If you want your body to function efficiently and effectively, there must be a balance between fasted and fed states. If you are constantly in either of these states, it will harm your health and wellbeing in the long run. The simplest way to ensure that this balance exists is through fasting.

Chapter 2: What is Intermittent Fasting 16/8?

Intermittent fasting is incredibly versatile. While following intermittent fasting, you can fast daily, on alternate days, or adjust the fasting protocol according to your needs and requirements. The most popular form of intermittent fasting is the 16/8 diet, also known as the 16:8 fasting diet or the lean gains method. This method of intermittent fasting was popularized by a trainer called Martin Berkhan. Here's a fun fact: did you know that Hugh Jackman followed the lean gains approach to achieve his famous Wolverine physique?

The 16/8 Protocol

This simple intermittent fasting protocol requires you to fast for sixteen hours daily. This automatically reduces the eating window to eight hours. If you take a moment and think about it, your body is regularly in a fasted state. Are you wondering how this happens? Well, as mentioned, your body is essentially fasting when you are asleep. Think of the 16/8 protocol as a mere extension of this fasted state. Perhaps the primary benefit of this form of intermittent fasting is its simplicity.

Most of us have busy lives and rushed mornings. If you are no stranger to skipping breakfast, this method will be quite easy to follow. It suggests that you fast for sixteen consecutive hours. According to your needs and requirements or convenience, you can change the fasting window. For instance, if you are comfortable with the idea of skipping breakfast or are used to doing this, then your first meal will be at noon and the last meal at eight in the evening. Do you see what happened here? You are automatically fasting for sixteen hours, and the eating window is restricted to eight hours. This is just one example of the lean gains protocol.

As mentioned earlier, you can customize the fast according to your obligations, lifestyle, and more. Let's say, if you like the idea of waking up early in the morning and exercising, you can reschedule the eating window to accommodate your nutritional needs after working out. For instance, you can wake up early in the morning, exercise, have your first meal at around 10 a.m. and the last at 6 p.m. As long as the eating window is restricted to eight hours, you can change the fasting schedule. This is entirely up to you. Intermittent fasting is not a restrictive diet; the only thing you need to pay attention to is when you eat.

During the eating window, you can consume three wholesome and healthy meals. You can also consume non-caloric foods and beverages during that window. As long as you don't over-compensate during the eating window by consuming unhealthy meals, you can achieve all the benefits of intermittent fasting. By following this protocol, your calorie intake will automatically be reduced. It also makes you more conscious about your eating patterns and dietary choices. A little extra attention and conscious effort are all it takes to achieve your weight loss and fitness goals. You will learn more in the upcoming chapters.

Cellular Changes

Now that you understand what intermittent fasting is, you need to understand how the process works on a cellular level. Several changes take place in your body while fasting. Your body is similar to a machine. All machines suffer from wear and tear when used regularly. Certain parts of the machine need to be replaced, the oil has to be changed, and it needs regular servicing. What happens to the machine without regular upkeep? Sooner or later, it will stop functioning. This is what happens to your body, too. A common mistake most of us make is we treat our bodies like tireless machines. To be fair, even machines need maintenance; the best way to improve your body's function is through intermittent fasting.

This dietary protocol triggers certain helpful changes at a cellular level through a process known as autophagy. In simple terms, autophagy is a natural process and is similar to regular servicing. It is triggered when your body is under stress; the word stress here doesn't have any negative connotations. Instead, it refers to the stress induced on the body during fasting when it needs to dip into its internal reserves of energy to keep functioning. Autophagy helps repair and replace damaged cells. In autophagy, your body starts to cannibalize all the old and defunct cells. It might sound morbid, but this is an incredibly helpful process. Without autophagy, there would be a buildup of defunct and malfunctioning cells in the body, which can hinder your overall wellbeing. This process is also known to remove the buildup of toxins. In a way, autophagy is like your body's housekeeping service; only when the damaged cells are removed or repaired can your body start to generate healthier ones. It helps detoxify your body from the inside.

Another essential cellular change pertains to the stabilization of blood sugar levels. Over the past few decades, diabetes has become a global health problem for millions of people. It is characterized by low levels of insulin and high levels of blood sugar. Your body produces the insulin hormone whenever you eat anything to process the food and convert it into glucose. Glucose levels in the blood increase when your body cannot produce sufficient insulin or if there's a resistance to it. All this is done away with when you don't eat anything. If you don't consume any food, your body doesn't have to produce insulin. It means you are reducing any fluctuations in blood sugar levels. As such, fasting may help reverse the effects of type-2 diabetes, however, always seek medical advice before trying any new diet, since people with diabetes may be at risk of hypoglycemia and hyperglycemia.

The human growth hormone (HGH) is crucial in regulating the body's metabolism. Fasting triggers the production of HGH. It not only regulates your metabolism but it promotes the development of muscles and bones and balances your body composition. Production of HGH typically reduces with age. Nevertheless, all this can be reversed by fasting.

In parallel, another important cellular change that occurs is the production of noradrenaline. This hormone is important in regulating your body's ability to burn fats. Since fats are the main source of energy during the absence of active food consumption, fat loss is one of the benefits of intermittent fasting. Coupled with noradrenaline production, this promotes weight loss and regulation in the long run.

As mentioned earlier, whenever you consume any food, only a portion is immediately used while the rest is stored in fat cells. Unless you stop eating, your body doesn't utilize these internal reserves of fats. Another cellular change that takes place is ketosis. Ketosis is not only natural but incredibly helpful, too. As you know, your body's primary source of energy is glucose whenever you consume food. Once all the glucose from the food you consume is used, your body actively starts looking for alternate energy sources. This is when the internal fat reserves are solicited. When your body dips into its internal reserves, fats are converted into energy molecules known as ketones, which quickly replace glucose as your primary source of energy. A wonderful thing about ketones is that ketone production isn't limited or reduced as long as there are sufficient reserves of fat present in the body. This stabilizes energy levels and keeps you going, even while fasting. Essentially, your body stays in ketosis as long as you don't consume any carbs or sugars. By increasing your intake of dietary fats and reducing the intake of unhealthy carbs and sugars, ketosis lasts for longer.

Myths about Intermittent Fasting

Intermittent fasting has become incredibly popular over recent years. Whenever something gains popularity, several misconceptions about it start circulating. In this section, we'll explore common myths about intermittent fasting and the corresponding facts. These myths can prevent you from attaining your weight loss and fitness goals, so being a little mindful is of the essence.

Myth #1: Small Meals Are Needed for Weight Loss

The most common myth about dietary protocols is that you need to consume small meals to promote and eventually trigger weight loss. If you're constantly eating, how can your body ever start burning fats? As mentioned, your body does not utilize its stored reserves unless you stop eating. Fasting reduces your insulin levels and promotes lipolysis, which is when your body starts burning its internal reserves of fats. If you constantly eat small meals, your body needs to expend a significant portion of its energy digesting the food you are consuming. Also, this increases blood sugar levels. All in all, small meals do not or rarely aid weight loss. If you want to lose weight and burn fats, you need to fast.

It's important to realize that your calorie intake will not magically be reduced with small meals. For instance, if you need to consume 2000 calories daily, you can eat three healthy and wholesome meals.

Whether they are three or six meals, the calorie intake doesn't change. Similarly, the energy expended by your body digesting these calories will also remain the same. Intermittent fasting promotes weight loss during its fasting window. During the eating window, you can schedule the meals according to your convenience, needs, goals, and more.

Myth #2: Skipping Breakfast is Harmful to Your Health

While following the intermittent fasting protocol, you can schedule it according to your usual lifestyle, habits, and daily requirements. If you are a breakfast eater, don't worry about skipping it. Similarly, if you don't like the idea of having breakfast, don't eat it. This should be the only consideration. Don't be under the misconception that skipping breakfast is necessarily harmful to one's health. In fact, if you think about it for a moment, the key to weight loss is reducing your calorie intake. There is no scientific evidence to support the claim that skipping breakfast can promote weight gain. So, you can stop worrying about weight gain whenever you skip breakfast. While fasting it is most important to schedule the meals so that they help satiate your appetite.

Myth #3: Intermittent Fasting Increases Nutritional Deficiencies

Intermittent fasting encourages you to fast daily. That said, it doesn't mean you are not eating food altogether. Instead, the eating window is restricted. Nutritional deficiencies occur when you don't pay attention to the type of foods you are consuming. By increasing your intake of wholesome and nutrient-dense ingredients, the chances of nutritional deficiencies are reduced. This is one reason you need to pay a lot of attention to the food choices you make, something most of us have complete control over. Go through the list of ingredients and food choices discussed in the next sections and the meal plan provided in this book to ensure your body gets all the nutrients it needs. If you are worried about any nutritional deficiencies, discuss them with your physician or healthcare provider. If needed, you can always opt for a nutrient supplement.

Myth #4: Intermittent Fasting Causes Eating Disorders

Intermittent fasting does not cause eating disorders. This is nothing more than a myth. If you eat a healthy diet and follow the fasting protocols to the letter, the chances of developing an eating disorder are almost non-existent. However, if you have a history of eating disorders (for example bulimia or anorexia) or are recovering from one, do not attempt fasting unless you have made a full recovery. Eating disorders arise when you go overboard and severely restrict your food intake. Rather than expose yourself to potentially harmful risks, eat until your body is full and always opt for healthy and wholesome ingredients.

Myth #5: Intermittent Fasting Can Cause Infertility

It's a popular misconception that fasting causes infertility in women. The hormonal changes in women's bodies are quite real, yet they don't result in any fertility issues. That said, if you are nursing, trying to conceive, or pregnant, fasting (or any other diet, for that matter) is not recommended. A woman's body is highly sensitive to signs of starvation. If your food intake is drastically reduced, your body may misinterpret it as starvation. Starvation can trigger hormonal imbalances. So, once again, it is important to pay attention to the food you are consuming and its quality.

Myth #6: Intermittent Fasting Can Result in Muscle Loss

People believe fasting results in muscle loss. As long as your body has internal reserves of energy to sustain itself and you consume healthy and wholesome meals during the eating window, you don't have to worry about muscle loss. Your body doesn't use muscle protein unless it has run out of all possible energy sources. So, starving is not a good idea. Intermittent fasting promotes weight loss without reducing your muscle mass. In fact, you can even increase your muscle mass by combining the protocol of intermittent fasting with a healthy diet and a good exercise routine.

Myth #7: Overeating Is a Common Side Effect of Intermittent Fasting

Regulating your appetite and making healthy dietary choices are two fundamental aspects of this diet that are well within your control. Overeating doesn't occur if you fill up on nutrient-dense and fiber-rich foods. During the first few days, your body is getting accustomed to intermittent fasting, and the chances of slightly overeating may increase. Once your body is used to fasting, this does not happen or rarely does. To reduce the risk of overeating, make sure you have intermittent fasting-friendly meals and snacks on hand. When delicious and nutritious meals are waiting for you, it becomes easier to eat healthily. Also, this reduces the urge to binge on sweet snacks and unhealthy junk food. Remind yourself that fasting doesn't have to be difficult—by changing your mindset about fasting and giving your diet a little conscious consideration, fasting becomes easy. You will learn more about doing all this in the subsequent chapters.

Myth #8: The Brain Needs a Constant Supply of Dietary Groups

People believe that abstaining from eating carbs every couple of hours will reduce their cognitive functioning. This is primarily based on the belief that your brain requires only glucose to support itself. In reality, the human body is quite resourceful and capable of adjusting and adapting to existing conditions. If you are not constantly eating carbs, your body produces glucose through a process known as gluconeogenesis. Even during a prolonged fast, your body produces sufficient ketones from its internal fat reserves. These ketones can fuel your brain and fulfill its glucose requirements. That said, if you feel lightheadedness or extreme fatigue after fasting, chances are you are not eating properly. It may also be a sign that your eating-fasting window schedule isn't suited to your needs and lifestyle.

In the end, you must let go of any misconceptions about intermittent fasting before you follow its protocols. Whether it is for your health or weight loss goals, intermittent fasting is incredibly effective when done right.

Chapter 3: The Benefits of Fasting

Intermittent fasting is growing popular these days, and for all the right reasons. Whether you want to lose weight and maintain weight loss or improve your overall health, intermittent fasting is a wonderful and accessible option. In this section, we'll look at all the various benefits of fasting.

Regulates Blood Sugar Levels

Whenever you consume any food, the pancreas secretes a hormone known as insulin. Insulin is essential in converting this food into glucose, an easily absorbable source of energy. Glucose is then transported to different cells across the body. Insulin is responsible for regulating your blood sugar levels. Type-2 diabetes has become a pandemic these days. It is a condition whereby your body is incapable of producing the insulin required to stabilize blood sugar levels (also known as insulin resistance). It occurs when your body starts developing immunity toward natural insulin secretion. Even though the pancreas does produce insulin, it is not the desired level to manage and balance blood sugar levels.

According to a study conducted by Terra G. Arnason et al. (2017), intermittent fasting can reduce blood sugar levels in individuals with type-2 diabetes. According to a review undertaken by Adrienne R. Barnosky et al. (2014), intermittent fasting reduces insulin resistance due to the automatic calorie reduction it engenders. So, even though you are not counting calories while following this diet, the benefits it offers don't go away.

By curbing insulin resistance, your body's sensitivity to insulin increases. This makes it easier for the glucose to circulate in the bloodstream and enter the cells more efficiently. This beneficial effect, combined with its blood sugar-reducing reaction, can help stabilize your blood sugar levels. As such, the risk of any spikes or crashes in blood sugar levels is significantly reduced. If you have type-2 diabetes it is recommended you seek medical advice before attempting intermittent fasting.

Tackles Inflammation

Your body's primary line of defense against the presence of any disease-causing pathogens or foreign bodies is inflammation. In limited amounts, inflammation is crucial for your overall health and wellbeing; it is a natural immune response. Usually, once the threat is neutralized, inflammation subsides. Unfortunately, when inflammation persists, it can manifest into a chronic health problem. In chronic inflammation, the immune system mistakenly attacks itself and other healthy cells, causing internal damage. It is also believed to be the precursor for several severe health conditions, including heart disease, rheumatoid arthritis, and even certain cancers.

According to the results obtained by a study conducted by Mo'ez Al-Islam E Faris et al. (2012), fasting regularly for an entire month can reduce inflammatory markers. These claims are also backed by another study conducted by Fehime B Aksungar et al. (2007). In an animal study conducted by In-Young Choi et al. (2016), any diet that mimics the eating patterns prescribed by fasting reduces inflammation. The researchers of this study believe this can help treat inflammatory conditions such as multiple sclerosis.

Stabilizes Blood Pressure and Cholesterol Levels

According to the 2017 report presented by The American Heart Association, heart disease accounted for around 31% of deaths globally, quite a startling and disturbing figure. The two common health markers associated with an increase in cardiovascular disorders are high cholesterol levels and high blood pressure. Shifting to intermittent fasting is a good idea to improve your heart health. According to a study conducted by Surabhi Bhutani et al. (2010), following intermittent fasting reduces blood triglycerides by 32% and cholesterol levels by 25%, all within eight weeks. In another study conducted on 110 obese adults by Biljana Beleslin et al. (2007), intermittent fasting seemed to reduce their levels of blood pressure, cholesterol, and triglycerides. By improving the primary markers associated with coronary disease, fasting can greatly improve your cardiovascular health.

Improves Cognitive Functioning

It turns out that ancient Greeks were onto something when they believed fasting could promote cognitive functioning. Remember the "food coma" discussed in the previous chapters? In truth, fasting has a powerful effect on brain health. According to Li Liao et al. (2013), fasting can improve the brain's structure and function. Though most of the research available in this aspect is from animal models, fasting seems to offer promising potential in improving brain health. In another study conducted by J. Lee et al. (2000), fasting promoted new neural cells in mice. Similarly, the results from a study by M. Tajes et al. (2010) indicated that intermittent fasting helped enhance cognitive functioning.

Promotes Weight Loss

One of the most compelling reasons why people turn to intermittent fasting is its great potential for weight loss. The primary concept of weight loss is the need for a calorie deficit. A calorie deficit occurs when your calorie intake is lower than calorie expenditure (in other words, you "burn" more than you eat). According to G. Zauner et al. (2000), short-term fasting increases the production of norepinephrine, a neurotransmitter believed to trigger weight loss by activating your body's internal fat-burning mechanism. According to a review by Grant M. Tinsley et al. (2015), intermittent fasting for 12-24 weeks could result in a significant decline in body fat and weight.

Another benefit of following intermittent fasting is it naturally promotes calorie restriction. The fact that your meal timings are restricted means the chances of mindlessly binging on foods are reduced. It also makes you more conscious of your body's hunger and satiety cues. A combination of these factors can help reduce your calorie consumption, provided you make healthy choices. Considering this approach, intermittent fasting is the ideal dieting protocol for weight loss and maintenance.

Stimulates Metabolism

Several hormones are secreted by your body to maintain your overall health and function. One hormone is the human growth hormone, or HGH. The production of this hormone naturally declines with age. Unfortunately, an HGH deficiency can have severe effects on your health.

According to research by A Juul et al. (1995), intermittent fasting promotes the production of growth hormones. HGH is essential for maintaining muscle strength, stamina, body temperature, kidney function, and weight management. According to a study conducted by N. Moller et al. (1991), it improves glucose metabolism in the body. In another study by Michael Hojby Rasmussen (2010), it was shown that a reduction in the production of HGH increases the risk of obesity. The simplest way to reverse it is by increasing the production of HGH.

According to a study conducted by B. Salgin et al. (2012), it was noticed that fasting for even 12 hours causes a significant increase in HGH production. These claims are supported by the findings of a study by M. L. Hartman et al. (1992), which suggests fasting increases HGH secretion. The levels of HGH can be further optimized when blood sugar and insulin levels are stabilized. Since intermittent fasting helps achieve this objective, it further increases the production of HGH.

Reduces the Risk of Cancer

According to animal and test-tube studies, intermittent fasting may also help prevent and improve the efficiency of treatments in tackling cancer. According to a study by Noeme Sousa Rocha et al. (2002), intermittent fasting can block the formation of tumors in rats. In another test-tube study conducted by Changhan Lee et al. (2013), intermittent fasting was shown to delay the growth of tumors. Lee and his research team noticed that regular fasting had a similar effect on cancerous cells as in chemotherapy. Their findings also suggest that intermittent fasting can improve the efficiency of chemotherapy drugs used to tackle cancer formation.

Although these results and findings are derived from animal studies, the potential offered by intermittent fasting cannot be disregarded. Despite these promising results, extensive research is still needed to fully understand how intermittent fasting can reduce the risks associated with cancer.

Kick-Starts Autophagy

As mentioned earlier, autophagy is a cellular change that occurs while fasting. This term refers to your body's internal mechanism responsible for cellular repair. In autophagy, the damaged cells are actively cannibalized by the healthy cells. Once the undesirable cells are all eliminated, it leaves room for more healthy and helpful cells to be produced. Self-cannibalization might sound worrisome, but it has a wonderful benefit. Over time, certain cells are damaged and may even cease to function altogether. These cells must be removed so your body can function optimally and create healthier cells again. This is where autophagy plays its role.

Easily Sustainable

Apart from all the different benefits mentioned so far, another advantage of intermittent fasting that cannot be overlooked is the convenience it offers. The 16/8 protocol is incredibly simple to follow and can be customized according to your needs and requirements. You can shift the fasting and eating windows according to your convenience, making it perfectly sustainable in the long run. Unlike most conventional diets, intermittent fasting doesn't place any restrictions on calorie counting or food restriction. Instead, it lets you eat to your heart's content, provided you don't consume any calories during the fasting window and opt for nutritional meals later.

Remember this: If you want to lose weight or improve your overall health, limit your intake of processed, prepackaged, and unhealthy foods. Rather than binge on unhealthy carbs and sugars and other foods devoid of nutrition, fill up on wholesome and

nutritious meals during the eating window. You can do all this without worrying about the calories you consume.

When you combine all the advantages offered by the 16/8 protocol, it becomes evident why it has become so incredibly popular.

Chapter 4: What to Know before Fasting

After going through the various benefits of intermittent fasting, chances are you are quite excited about getting started. This customizable and sustainable diet is ideal for all healthy adults, but everything has its limitations. This section will look at a few important considerations you need to keep in mind before embarking on this diet.

Who Shouldn't Try Fasting?

If you fall into any of the categories mentioned in the section, refrain from fasting.

Fasting is neither ideal nor encouraged for pregnant women. The nutritional requirements of a pregnant woman differ from the needs of others. Your body not only has to sustain itself but support the fetus as well. While fasting is safe for most, attempting any form of diet during pregnancy is not recommended. To date, there is no scientific evidence to fully determine the effects of fasting on an unborn infant. That said, it is a common belief that fasting can

disrupt your nutritional intake and, in turn, affect the nutritional needs of the fetus.

Aside from pregnant women, if you are breastfeeding, you should not attempt fasting or any diet for that matter. Once again, your body's requirements at this time are quite different, and right now, your primary focus should only be on taking care of yourself and the baby. Fasting can wait a few months. A woman's body is quite sensitive to signals of starvation. Even if fasting is a voluntary choice, your body cannot distinguish between starvation and a voluntary fast. Whenever this happens, your body's primary focus shifts to its survival. This survival instinct prevents all other non-essential functions in favor of survival, such as reproduction. If you are trying to conceive, avoid fasting or making any drastic changes to your regular diet.

If you have any preexisting health conditions, or liver or kidney troubles, fasting is not advised. If you suffer from bouts of weakness, are malnourished, or anemic, fasting is not recommended at all. Before you start fasting, consider seeing your healthcare provider for their medical opinion. Similarly, certain medications should never be taken while fasting. If you use medicines to regulate your blood pressure, treat a weak immune system or due to poor blood circulation, avoid fasting altogether. If you want to try your hand at fasting, make sure to consult your healthcare provider beforehand.

If you are recovering from an eating disorder or have a history of eating disorders, attempting any diet, even intermittent fasting, is not advisable. Whether it is bulimia or anorexia or any other eating disorder, your body needs a while to recover from the condition. So, unless you are 100% recovered and your doctor has cleared you for fasting, don't try it.

If you are recovering from an illness, have recently undergone major surgery, or are preparing for major surgery, avoid fasting. Following a diet that restricts the eating window during these periods is not recommended. Your primary nutritional

requirements differ during the recovery period, and fasting can harm this process. You can start fasting once you have fully recovered. Once again, do not forget to consult your physician or dietitian before attempting this diet.

Fasting is not encouraged for children. Occasional fasting for short periods will not harm them, yet a long-term fasting protocol is far from ideal. A child's body requires plenty of nutrition to grow healthily and sustain itself. Your child's pediatrician must approve the diet before you make any drastic changes to it. According to certain laws and provisions in the United States, it is illegal for a child to fast. By contrast, obese children are allowed to fast under adult supervision and a doctor's guidance in Europe, provided the child does so voluntarily.

All healthy adults can fast without any major worries. Fasting regularly cleanses your system from the inside, and there are no reasons why a healthy adult should abstain from fasting. Among several benefits already listed, fasting regulates the levels of blood sugar.

Remember, before making any dietary changes, don't forget to consult your healthcare provider.

Considerations before Fasting

The 16/8 protocol is incredibly simple and doesn't require any drastic lifestyle changes. Apart from your state of health, there are three simple considerations you need to remember before starting this diet. The first consideration is your personal opinion about fasting. The second one is your daily schedule, and the third, your regular diet. These three factors may sound unimportant, but they are in fact crucial for determining your motivation while following intermittent fasting.

While making dietary changes may sound simple, a significant change in your body and mind is required. Unless you have an open mind about fasting, starting intermittent fasting can be tricky. Remember, you need to restrict the eating window to only eight hours daily. This means you need to fast for sixteen hours. Unless you are mentally prepared for the diet, making this change will prove extremely difficult. Your personal opinion about fasting also determines your level of investment in the diet. Ensure that you are comfortable with the idea of fasting and that it does not become a source of additional stress. We already lead busy and hectic lifestyles, and diet must not be a source of added stress or a burden. Take time and carefully consider how this protocol works. Unless you are completely comfortable with the idea of fasting, do not attempt it. If doubts persist, you are only increasing the chances of giving up on this diet. This may, in turn, demotivate you from attempting to fast in the future. If you want to fast and are genuinely interested, keep an open mind and work on changing your mindset.

Evidently, your regular diet plays a significant role in your life. Take time and carefully consider what your usual diet looks like. If it is predominantly made up of processed foods, carbs, sugars, and other prepackaged foods, shifting to this new diet will take a good deal of time. Believe it or not, a diet rich in carbs and sugar is rather addictive. Your mindset aside, you need to gradually condition your body to the idea of depriving it of food temporarily. If you've never fasted before and this is your first attempt, take a little extra time.

While shifting to this diet is simple, you need to be patient. For instance, if you are used to constantly snacking or consuming high-calorie foods, slowly increase the amount of time between two meals and reduce the number of snacks you consume. Another simple suggestion to make the transition easier is to replace carbs and processed foods with nutrient-dense and wholesome ingredients.

The third consideration is your usual schedule or lifestyle. Intermittent fasting is not complicated and offers great flexibility, unlike other dietary protocols. That said, you cannot follow a diet if it clashes with or somehow impedes your regular schedule. For instance, if you are in the habit of skipping breakfast, following this protocol becomes all the more simple. Similarly, if you like the idea of waking up early in the morning and getting in a good workout, shift the eating window accordingly. Regardless of your daily lifestyle, intermittent fasting can be customized with a little conscious thought and planning.

You must spend time carefully thinking about all these considerations; after all, your chances of sticking to this diet depend on them.

Chapter 5: Understanding Weight Loss Differences between Men and Women

A factor commonly blamed for weight gain is a slow metabolism. Chances are, you've heard this phrase tossed around in casual conversations. What does "metabolism" really mean, and what role does it play in weight loss? Let us answer these two questions in this chapter to explain the difference between weight loss in men and women.

Understanding Body Metabolism

Several processes are constantly working behind the scenes in your body. From respiration to digestion, hormone regulation, growth and repair of cells, and blood circulation, every system in your body requires energy to function efficiently. These functions tend to go on in the background even when you are resting. In reality, none of these processes ever stop. Most of these involuntary functions are crucial for your wellbeing and health. So, where does this energy come from? Simply put, the metabolism is the primary process that enables your body to transform the food you consume into energy.

During metabolism, the calories in the food you consume mingle with oxygen in the bloodstream and are transformed into the energy your body needs to function.

This process is known as metabolism or basal metabolic rate. Different factors determine your basal metabolic rate. The most common factors to pay attention to are sex, age, body size, and composition. Those with more developed muscles or a larger body tend to have more calories they can burn even while resting. Calorie burning is reduced as you age because the amount of muscle present in the body tends to diminish while fat increases. Sex also plays a significant role when it comes to your body's metabolism. From a biological point of view, men tend to have more muscle and less fat than women of the same age and weight. This is one of the reasons why men tend to burn more calories than women.

Beyond all these factors, your body's main functions and the energy it needs is fairly constant. Two additional factors determine the calories you burn daily, namely thermogenesis and physical activity. As mentioned earlier, the food you eat is transformed into energy by your body. Whenever you eat, the food is first digested, then absorbed, transported, and a portion of it is stored before it is assimilated and expelled. This entire process is known as thermogenesis.

Simply put, it is nothing more than food processing. Only about 10% of the calories obtained from the proteins and carbs you consume are used during digestion and food absorption. Physical activity in all its forms and exercise account for the number of calories your body burns daily.

Now that you understand what metabolism is and the factors that influence it, let's explore the relationship between metabolism and weight. A fairly common assumption is that your metabolism is to blame for weight gain. Since metabolism is a natural and essential process for survival, several mechanisms are in place to regulate it and ensure all its needs are fulfilled. Excessive weight gain due to a metabolic problem is not common; this usually occurs when the thyroid gland is underactive or subject to conditions such as Cushing's syndrome. Weight gain is not as simple as this. Instead, it is a severely complicated process. It is the culmination of genetic and hormonal makeup and composition, diet, as well as your daily lifestyle and environment. Should there be an imbalance in any of these factors, it will cause an imbalance in the whole system; for instance, if you eat more calories than your body burns, the result will be weight gain.

It is true some people can lose weight more quickly than others. If you want to lose weight, you must make sure your body burns more calories than you consume. No one is exempt from this rule. By devising a diet that causes an energy deficit or increases the calories burned during the day, you can lose weight.

You might not have much control over how quickly the basal metabolic rate works, but you can regulate the number of calories burned through physical activity. The more physically active you are, the greater the calories burned. This is one reason why fasting increases your body's metabolism by promoting the calories burned during the fasting period. The simplest and most efficient way to burn calories is through aerobic ("cardio") activities such as jogging, walking, cycling, or yoga. Even engaging in thirty minutes of physical activity daily can significantly increase your calorie expenditure.

If you have specific fitness or weight loss goals, the level of physical activity required may be higher. If you cannot exercise for half-an-hour, you can break it down into ten-minute intervals and include them into your daily routine. Besides aerobic activities, strength training exercises such as weightlifting, help to build your muscles while reducing the fatty tissues present within. What does all this mean? Essentially, that all the extra movement increases calorie expenditure.

Weight Loss in Men and Women

You might have heard that men are from Mars while women are from Venus. This popular book on relationships explains the differences between how men and women communicate, express their emotions, and behave in general. There is another aspect of life where women and men differ: how the metabolism works for weight loss.

Previously, women were primarily interested in losing weight and maintaining a thin physique due to social or cultural pressure more than health concerns (at least in Western societies). Men were primarily focused on building muscles, taking supplements, and enhancing their muscles. Nowadays, a shift has occurred in what men and women are trying to achieve. Both genders are now more focused on reducing fat while maintaining a leaner physique. However, there are a couple of differences between the sexes due to our genetic coding. This section will look at all the different factors that result in varying weight loss for men and women.

From a strictly genetic standpoint, men have more muscle mass and less fat than women. This difference is due to higher levels of testosterone in men. This is why their calorie consumption is typically higher than women's to maintain muscle mass and body weight. Suppose you compare two individuals with similar body weight, but one has more muscle mass than the other. In that case, the person with greater muscle mass requires more calories to sustain their weight because their calorie expenditure is higher. Muscle tends to burn more calories than fat does, even at rest. A general notion is that around 3500 calories are required for one pound of muscle mass. Whenever you are trying to lose weight, only about half of the weight loss is from muscles. By concentrating on what you eat and including strength training, you can considerably minimize muscle loss. Usually, both men and women start losing muscle mass during their thirties. In parallel, loss of muscle also affects the immune system and mobility.

How we carry our body weight is also quite different based on which gender we are. If men gain a little weight, the primary area where it goes is the abdomen. This explains why most men are "apple-shaped." On the other hand, premenopausal women tend to put on weight near the hips and less in the abdominal region. Due to hormonal changes during menopause, post-menopausal women usually gain weight in the abdominal region because of a reduction in estrogen.

Regardless of gender, any excess fat that starts accumulating in the abdominal area and around the organs bears significant health risks. This is known as visceral fat, which is highly inflammatory. This unhealthy fat is directly associated with an increased risk of cardiovascular disorders, fatty liver disease, and diabetes. In contrast, the soft fat present directly under the skin isn't metabolically dangerous and is responsible for regulating your body temperature and overall state of health.

This brings us to another important notion about weight loss, which states that men can lose weight more easily than women. A popular theory is associated with the role of hormones and the brain's response to calorie restriction. From an evolutionary point of view, a woman's body is genetically designed for reproduction. This activity requires significant energy. Whenever the brain notices a reduction in energy available, it tends to divert all the available resources for life-sustaining activities, and reproduction is not one of them. This is one reason why excessive calorie restriction in women causes irregularities in menstrual cycles and might also lead to fertility issues. All in all, a woman's body needs a greater percentage of body fat when compared to a man.

These differences in body fat percentage are all a part of our basic physiology. Men tend to have a weight-loss edge over women due to their elevated testosterone levels and low levels of estrogen.

On average, women tend to have anywhere between 6-11% more body fat than men. From puberty to menopause, even when women consume fewer calories than men, their average body fat level is higher. Now, it is important to understand that fat isn't always synonymous with unhealthiness. Even if women have larger fat stores, this does not necessarily mean extra weight. If a woman has 10% more body fat than a man, it doesn't mean she is 10% "fatter." A perfectly fit and healthy woman will have 6-11% more body fat than a healthy man.

This basic difference in physiology, coupled with how fats are stored in the body, results in differences in weight loss. As mentioned earlier, fats in men accumulate in the abdominal region while fats tend to be more spread out in women. So, the weight loss is more noticeable and visible in men than women because of how the internal reserves of fats are stored. Despite differences in weight loss between men and women, these tend to even out in the long run. Even if women are better at storing fats, their body's ability to burn more fat during exercise is higher than men.

In the end, weight loss is an achievable and maintainable goal for adult men and women alike. Forget about your gender, and instead shift your attention toward leading a healthier life, exercising regularly, and consuming a healthy diet. Once you do all this, weight loss and maintenance become easy, regardless of whether you are a woman or a man.

Chapter 6: How to Exercise While Fasting

Intermittent fasting and regular exercise are the simplest ways to improve your overall health while attaining fitness and weight loss goals. When it comes to weight loss and muscle gain, calories are not the only factors that play an important role; exercise also helps hormone optimization. By combining these two aspects, attaining your fitness and health goals becomes easier and more manageable. A combination of exercise and diet aids the production of growth hormones and increases insulin sensitivity.

It is rather unfortunate that most people obsess over the calories they consume and spend. Some are also worried about muscle loss. Muscle loss occurs only when you exercise without refueling your body. By understanding the positive effects of exercise on the hormones in your body during the fasting state, you'll realize that fasting improves muscle health and promotes fat loss at the same time.

If you are worried about exercising on an empty stomach, it's time to put these fears to rest! It is not only okay to exercise on an empty stomach, but it increases the benefits of exercise as well. Intermittent fasting is simply an extension of the period your body goes without food, including the time you sleep. The fasting window stretches the last bite of food you consumed, until you eat again. As such, the ideal time to work out is after you wake up in the morning. This works with your body's internal circadian rhythm (which regulates sleep) and boosts the benefits of working out.

Exercise Options

If you are eager to add exercise into your daily routine, here are the best, true and tested options to go for.

Cardio

Cardio is a form of aerobic activity that engages different muscle groups in your body. Whether it is walking, running, jogging, biking or swimming, these are all examples of aerobic activities. The hormonal benefits of exercising during a fasted state are associated with depletion of glycogen stored in the muscles and liver. You can indulge in cardio while fasting, but your overall performance throughout depends on your body's stage of fat adaptation. Fat adaptation refers to a state whereby your body no longer depends on glycogen to support itself and instead concentrates on burning the internal reserves of fat to fuel its energy requirements.

Invariably, it will take your body some time to get used to the new diet. During the initial days, you may notice a dip in your usual performance. Once your body is used to burning fats, your performance is bound to improve. If you are exercising in a fasted state, don't forget to refuel after the exercise. Otherwise, it increases the risk of starvation. Finally, it is very important to note that if your body shifts to a state of starvation, it stops burning fats and instead hoards all calories to sustain itself.

Sprint Training

High-intensity interval training (HIIT), also known as sprint training, involves short bursts of exercise followed by a period of rest or recovery. A typical HIIT workout lasts anywhere between

15-30 minutes. This form of exercise is time-efficient and offers health benefits that surpass those of traditional aerobic exercises. HIIT can increase your strength, stamina, promote cognitive function, increase growth hormones, and improve your body composition. Sprint training can be easily incorporated into your intermittent fasting schedule. To maximize the benefits of this exercise, make sure that you stay in the fasted state for at least two hours after exercising.

Lifting Weights

Lifting weights helps develop and strengthen the muscles, increase stamina, and build lean body fat. Lifting weights in a fasted state is fine. However, you need to pay a little attention to the role of glucose. After lifting weights, your muscles need additional glucose to repair and restore themselves. In a fasted state, your body first depletes the available reserves of glycogen (stored glucose) before moving on to burning fats. If your workout includes lifting weights, you can do so even in a fasted state, but you need to refuel your body once the workout is over. Unlike sprint training, lifting weights increases the stress on your body. As with cardio, you will need a while to increase your body's ability to power through a full weightlifting session. You may notice a decline in your endurance during the phase of adaptation; once your body turns on its internal fat-burning mechanism, exercising becomes easier. So, if you want to lift weights, make sure that you do so after eating.

Exercise Tips

Before you start exercising on the 16/8 protocol, bear in mind the following.

The first thing you need to consider is the timing of the exercise. If you've never attempted fasting before, it will be a significant change for your body to adapt to. To facilitate the transition and improve the workout's efficiency while fasting, you need to decide when you want to exercise. You can exercise before, after, or during the eating window.

The 16/8 protocol is one of the most popular methods of intermittent fasting. Suppose you believe your overall performance while exercising is superior on an empty stomach. In that case, you can exercise before the eating window. If you don't like the idea of exercising on an empty stomach, then do it during the eating window. The same rule applies to anyone who wants to capitalize on nutrition after working out. Performance and recovery are usually optimized after your body has sufficient fuel available. For instance, if you are lifting weights or performing cardio, you must refuel your body afterward. For these exercises, the ideal time is to exercise on an empty stomach right before the fasting window ends. This allows you to refuel your body, promote muscle development and stimulate fat loss.

Another important consideration to remember is the type of workout you opt for according to your macronutrient intake. Pay attention to the macros you consume in a day before you exercise, and anytime you eat later is important. For instance, cardio or high-intensity interval training can be performed even if your carbohydrate intake is low. By contrast, you need a significantly higher amount of carbs in your system to power through a strength training session.

To build and maintain muscle mass, it's not just important to exercise—you need to pay attention to the diet, too. If this is your main motivation for exercising, you need to make sure you consume food immediately after working out. One of the major advantages of combining intermittent fasting and exercise is that you get a chance to time the workout during the eating window, so your body gets all the nutrients it needs. Once again, you need to consume carbs and proteins in sufficient amounts after heavy lifting to promote muscle regeneration and muscle development. If you are indulging in any strength training, you need to consume around 20 grams of carbs and proteins within one hour of exercising.

Now that you're aware of all these dietary considerations, here are a few tips you can use to promote the efficiency of your exercise regimen and weight loss.

As established, meal timing is crucial when it comes to exercising. During high-intensity or moderate-intensity workouts, you need to eat something close to the workout schedule. This ensures your body has sufficient glycogen to power through the workout. For these exercises, the ideal time is after the eating window ends.

It isn't just food that matters when it comes to exercise. In fact, you need to ensure thorough hydration. Fasting doesn't mean you don't drink any water; if you are dehydrated, it increases stress on the muscles and reduces your workout efficiency. It also increases the risk of burning out. In parallel, you must also maintain your electrolyte levels. A good source of hydration helps replenish your electrolytes and is low in calories. That said, drinking Gatorade, Powerade, or any other sports drink loaded with sugars during the fasting window is not recommended.

During the initial days of shifting to intermittent fasting, your energy levels will fluctuate. In this transition period, you need to be extremely patient; there's no point in rushing into high-intensity training when your energy levels are low or wavering. Once your body is accustomed to the new fasting schedule, your energy levels will stabilize, making it easier to work out efficiently. During the initial period, any form of gentle exercises such as walking, yoga, Pilates, and jogging will suffice. Take it at your pace.

Last but definitely not least, one thing you should never forget is to listen to your own body's cues. The human body is quite smart, and it knows what it needs. If you feel weak or dizzy, it can be a sign of dehydration or low blood sugar levels. If so, stop exercising and have a carbohydrate and electrolyte mix immediately. If you are too tired to exercise, pay attention to your body's needs and requirements. Unless you take good care of it, it cannot function, much less actively or efficiently. Before you start any exercise regimen, don't forget to consult your healthcare provider or a professional trainer. This is especially true if you have any preexisting health conditions that can affect your mobility.

Chapter 7: Beginning the 16/8 Fasting Diet

Congratulations on making it this far! By now, you are aware of the various benefits intermittent fasting offers. Shifting to this diet immediately might be tempting, but a little planning and preparation are needed before you make any changes. In this insightful chapter, you will be introduced to simple dietary suggestions and steps you can follow to get started on the 16/8 diet.

What to Eat During the Fasting Window

The only rule to remember during the fasting window is that you should not consume any calories. If you consume calories, your body shifts from a fast to a fed state. That said, it doesn't mean you cannot drink any calorie-free beverages. In this section, let's look at a couple of options you can safely consume during the fasting window.

Apple Cider Vinegar

One of the best things you can consume during the fasting window without any worries is apple cider vinegar. Apple cider vinegar helps stabilize the electrolyte levels, reduces hunger pangs and rebalances pH levels in the digestive tract. Apple cider vinegar is known to have anti-inflammatory and antibacterial properties that help strengthen your immune system and promote proper digestive functioning. Moreover, it gives your metabolism a quick boost, which is much needed for burning fats efficiently. Apple cider vinegar also contains essential minerals such as potassium, magnesium, and iron, all good for your health.

Baking Soda

While it is commonly used in cooking, you may be surprised to learn that you can drink baking soda! Your body's internal pH tends to change during the fasting period. Drinking a little baking soda helps restore this pH balance. It also alleviates tiredness, making you feel more energetic. Add a teaspoon of food-grade baking soda to a glass of water and drink it during the fasting period to keep hunger pangs or cravings at bay. Sodium bicarbonate or baking soda replenishes any lost sodium during the fasting period. As mentioned, ketosis can have a diuretic effect, which means your body starts to lose its internal reserves of sodium and water. Baking soda helps neutralize this while keeping you hydrated.

Herbal Teas

Sipping on herbal teas is an efficient and delicious way to tackle hunger pangs during the fasting period. Simply make sure that you do not add any sugar, sweeteners, or honey to your cup of herbal tea. A freshly brewed cup of peppermint tea can re-energize and refresh your mind, whereas chamomile tea has a calming and soothing effect. Depending on what you are in the mood for, sip on a cup of freshly brewed herbal tea to feel better. You can also drink unsweetened green tea; it is rich in antioxidants that tackle inflammation and promote your body's metabolism to burn fats efficiently.

Glauber's Salt

Taking Glauber's salt or sodium sulfate decahydrate is an excellent way to boost your metabolism while making it easier to get through the fasting period. It also helps to stabilize your electrolyte levels and prevent dehydration. Glauber's salt is safe for daily consumption. That said, do not consume more than 20 grams of salts on any given day. Add a teaspoon of the salt to a glass of water and drink it whenever you are fasting. These salts act as mild laxatives and improve digestion while relieving uncomfortable symptoms of constipation. So, consuming too much of these salts can result in diarrhea.

Coffee

Coffee is a great way to suppress hunger while fasting. It not only gives you an instant boost of energy but also helps to stabilize your blood sugar levels and promote fat utilization. If the eating window starts at noon, you can start your day with a cup of black coffee. Once again, you mustn't add any milk, creamer, sugar, or any other sweetener to your cup of coffee. You can, however, add a pinch of cinnamon or cocoa powder to give your morning coffee a more interesting profile. Remember, coffee is a natural diuretic, and consuming too much of it can quickly dehydrate you. Excess caffeine can trigger anxiety, increase stress, and disrupt your sleeping pattern. Avoid consuming coffee past 8 p.m. in the evening. In parallel, make sure you drink sufficient water to keep your body hydrated and well-lubricated.

Consuming these calorie-free beverages during your fasting period makes it easier to stamp out any hunger pangs. Most of these healthy options assist the beneficial cellular changes triggered by fasting.

How to Break a Fast

As mentioned in the previous chapter, you need to slowly get your body accustomed to fasting for prolonged periods following the 16/8 protocol. Since you will be fasting daily, how you break your fast is of utmost importance.

Fasting may sound simple, especially in the initial stages when your motivation is quite high. Unless you plan for it, following this diet will become tricky in the long run. Reduce the chances of giving up on this diet by letting go of an "I can wing it" mentality. You need a proper plan of action if you want to improve your overall health and fitness levels. "Failing to plan is planning to fail"— remember this mantra in all aspects of your life!

As we've seen, several changes occur in your body during the fasting window. One of the most important changes is ketosis. The liver produces ketones to sustain you, which can increase the stress on your digestive system. So, breaking your fast properly is crucial in managing the stress on your digestive system. Excess stress can trigger inflammation and induce other complications. This further worsens when you consume unhealthy and processed foods rich in carbs and sugars. Inflammation is also a primary cause of weight gain. It also harms your immune system.

If you don't have a well-designed plan in place, chances are you will eat the first thing you can get your hands on after breaking the fast. You need to avoid certain foods, especially those rich in carbs, since this increases sodium retention. The chances of gaining weight spike when there is excess sodium present in the body. Remember, your body eliminates sodium during fasting. Binging on carbs reverses this process, triggering anti-diuresis that causes bloating. Apart from this, it can also reduce your energy levels.

Here is one reason you need to pay extra attention to how you end the fast. One of the best ways to end the fast is by consuming a little apple cider vinegar. It helps to restore the pH level in your gut, neutralizes harmful bacteria in the digestive tract, and regulates your blood sugar levels. Since it is a calorie-free ingredient, you can also consume it during the fasting period. However, the best time to have apple cider vinegar is as soon as you start the fast. If the taste of raw apple cider vinegar is off-putting, you can add a pinch of cinnamon and squeeze half a lime into a glass of water. To stabilize your electrolyte levels, don't hesitate to add a pinch of sea salt as well. Sip on this mixture for thirty minutes before breaking the fast. Alternatively, you can end the fast by drinking a glass of warm water mixed with a little honey and lemon juice. The citric acid stimulates the digestive enzymes and "warms up" your gut for the food you will eat after fasting.

Another healthy option is to drink a little bone broth. Bone broth is a superfood rich in electrolytes and essential nutrients your body needs. It also stimulates the production of digestive enzymes and facilitates the absorption of nutrients from the food you will consume later. While fasting, your body is in self-cleanse mode, and it needs a while to get used to digesting and absorbing food once you start eating. This is one reason you need to pay extra attention to what you eat after ending the fast. Likewise, you can drink vegetable broth, organic soups, or anything else easily digested. This simple habit reduces the chances of overeating or binging on unhealthy foods.

What to Eat Right after Breaking the Fast

Again, and this can never be stressed enough, it will take time to get used to fasting daily. Apart from preparing your body to break the fast, paying attention to what you eat after the fast ends is equally important. If you don't want to undo all the benefits of fasting, consuming a well-balanced diet is crucial.

If you end the fast by consuming foods rich in carbs and sodium, it increases water retention, which will result in weight gain. Since intermittent fasting's primary aim is weight loss, you must avoid foods that increase water retention. Your body needs to secrete insulin to transport the essential nutrients from one cell to another. A drastic spike in insulin levels, which occurs when you consume carbon sugars, can induce lethargy and drowsiness. So, make sure that the first meal you consume after breaking the fast has a low glycemic index. Meals like these help your body to stay in a semi-fasted state for longer and reduce blood sugar level fluctuations.

Don't worry about self-cannibalization of muscles if your body stays in ketosis for a while longer. This does not occur unless your body has thoroughly exhausted all the sources of energy at its disposal. If you follow the protocols of intermittent fasting properly, you will not shift into starvation mode. Eating a handful of nuts, eggs, spinach, and healthy fats, such as avocados, is an example of a low glycemic meal.

Another healthy option for ending your fast is eating fresh fruit. Fructose is the natural sugar present in fruit, which can be easily metabolized by the liver. This also helps replenish the depleted stores of glycogen. The liver can store anywhere between 100-150 grams of glycogen. While fasting, the glycogen reserves are exhausted before it starts burning fats. To replace the lost glycogen, eat fresh fruit. Fruit is also rich in nutrients and vitamins your body needs to function optimally. If you consume foods with a high glycemic index after breaking the fast, it will undo all your fasting efforts. Any foods rich in glycogen will increase fat accumulation. Ideally, opt for foods rich in fiber and low in sugar, such as berries, apples, and melons.

There are no dietary restrictions or calorie considerations you need to worry about while following the 16/8 protocol. However, this is no excuse to go overboard and binge on unhealthy foods. Since the eating window stretches over eight hours, you have ample time to consume all the calories your body needs. Ideally, the first meal should be no more than 500 calories. In reality, it becomes far easier to make sure your body gets all the nutrients it needs by planning your meals in advance. If you exercise before the fasting window ends, make sure you consume food that replenishes your glycogen stores.

The good news is, you don't have to spend hours on end searching for intermittent fasting-friendly recipes. All the recipes you need are provided in this book. Carefully go through them, select the ones that appeal to you, and create a meal plan accordingly. Once you have all the ingredients purchased and prepped, cooking becomes easier and more enjoyable. You'll be compelled to make healthier and more conscious food choices as well.

Basic Dietary Suggestions

In this section, we'll take a look at the different foods you can consume after your fast ends without worrying. All these options are rich in nutrients that your body needs and aid weight loss.

Leafy Vegetables

All leafy vegetables, including kale, spinach, Swiss chard, amaranth, and rosella, abound with antioxidants and various vitamins and minerals. They are also low in calories and rich in dietary fiber. Leafy greens are the perfect addition to any diet.

Fish

Fish is a phenomenal source of lean protein and heart-healthy Omega-3 fatty acids. Naturally fatty fish such as trout, sardines, salmon, mahi-mahi, and cod are superb options. You can consume anywhere between 5-8 ounces of fish daily without any worries. The Omega-3 fatty acids and other helpful nutrients found in fish can improve your cognitive functioning and cardiovascular health. Apart from that, they're quite easy on the digestive system, too. Whenever you choose to eat fish, opt for the ones caught in the wild instead of factory-farmed fish.

Legumes

Legumes are a great source of digestive fiber, vitamins, and nutrients that your body needs. All the digestive fiber present in legumes promotes digestion and better absorption of nutrients. Legumes are incredibly diverse, vegan-friendly, and a healthy source of carbohydrates. They can easily and safely be incorporated into any meal. The fiber found in legumes increases satiety without added calories, which is crucial in intermittent fasting; when your hunger is satiated, getting through the fasting window becomes easier.

Avocados

One of the best sources of healthy and natural dietary fats is avocado. Avocados are a superfood loaded with Omega 3 fatty acids and digestive fiber, and are a great source of health-boosting protein. From smoothies and whole wheat toasts to salads, avocados can be easily incorporated into your daily meals.

Probiotics

Did you know that your gut harbors millions of bacteria known as the "gut microbiome?" Don't worry, as not all types of bacteria are harmful. In fact, certain types of bacteria are desirable to promote digestion and absorption of nutrients. When the gut microbiome functions properly, your digestive health improves. It also reduces the risk of inflammation. The simplest way to feed the gut microbiome is by adding probiotics into your daily diet. Probiotics are live microorganisms that promote the health of the gut microbiome, and the most common types are fermented foods such as yogurt, kombucha, buttermilk, kimchi, and sauerkraut. Instead of the store-bought variants filled with additives, try to make these at home with simple ingredients.

Berries

There are countless types of berries to choose from, and they're all rich in vitamin A and C and several antioxidants. They are also low in calories. Different berries you can consume without any worries are raspberries, strawberries, blueberries, blackberries, and even cherries. You can add them to smoothies or even turn them into a guilt-free dessert. The antioxidants reverse oxidative stress, fight free radicals, and regulate inflammation. Berries are also believed to strengthen the immune system. Whether fresh or frozen, berries are bound to be a wonderful and tasty addition to your daily diet.

Whole Foods

Make it a point to consciously add healthier whole foods (brown bread, pasta, rice, etc.) to your diet instead of the processed variants. Whole foods are rich in dietary fibers and several nutrients good for overall health. They also improve your body's metabolism, digestive health, and help maintain satiety.

Healthy Carbs

Just because intermittent fasting doesn't impose strict dietary rules doesn't mean you should binge on unhealthy carbs. For instance, eating a bag of chips or a candy bar at the end of the fasting window does not do you any favors. Unhealthy carbs are rich in empty calories without any added nutrients. Instead, opt for low-carb fruits and vegetables.

Eggs

Eggs are a great source of protein and dietary fats. Consume at least two eggs daily to improve your health. They also have a low glycemic index and contain nutrients, so ending your fast by eating eggs is an accessible option. Eggs are low in calories, easy to cook, and very versatile.

Apart from all these foods, don't forget to drink sufficient water. You need to drink at least eight glasses (around two liters) of water daily. Water helps flush out any toxins present within the body in the dissolved fat. Whenever you make any dietary changes, hydration should be your priority. You can even add a sprig of fresh mint leaves or a couple of slices of lemon or cucumber to spruce up regular water and make it more interesting.

Getting Started with Intermittent Fasting

Now that you have all the information about intermittent fasting, it's time to get started. In this section, let's look at simple steps you can follow to successfully transition into the 16/8 intermittent fasting protocol.

Start with the Groundwork

The first step of shifting to intermittent fasting is to complete the required groundwork. Essentially, you need to carefully consider your usual schedule and lifestyle. Once you have a rough routine in place, determine the ideal timing for fasting. If you are used to waking up early in the morning and exercising, the fasting window will be quite different than for someone who prefers skipping breakfast. This first step is important because it determines whether the diet is sustainable in the long run. Carefully go through all the aspects covered until now, and it will become easy to determine how you wish to go about this diet.

Get the Tools Required

Don't be afraid to experiment with your diet. You can start with a specific fasting and eating routine and then shift to something else if you realize it isn't working. The process of trial and error is incredibly helpful when it comes to this protocol of intermittent fasting. In parallel, you will need plenty of recipes to design a meal plan that's ideal for intermittent fasting. All the recipes you need to create a detailed meal plan have been included in this book. Go through the recipes, put together a meal plan, and start batch cooking over the weekends to save time during the week.

While making a dietary change, pay special attention to what you are eating. The simplest way to do this is by keeping a food journal or using a mobile app to track what you eat. This is not the same as counting calories; the simple act of writing down your food choices makes you more conscious and allows you to make healthier choices in the future. This also helps you understand which foods work well with your metabolism.

Time to Transition

Shifting to intermittent fasting should not be a decision taken on a whim. If you want this diet to be sustainable, planning is needed. Take time, consider when you want to start this diet, and make a note of it. To transition into this diet, there are certain helpful changes you can make. For instance, if your usual diet is rich in carbs, slowly start cutting them down. If you are used to snacking constantly, stop snacking between meals and slowly increase the duration between two meals. By making these simple changes, controlling your hunger and shifting to intermittent fasting becomes easier. In a way, you are conditioning your body and mind to the idea of fasting daily. If you want, you can fast for brief periods daily to see how you feel about it and how your body responds.

Support System

Never underestimate the importance of having a support system in your life. Be it your friends, family members, coworkers, or other loved ones, they can all be a part of your support system. Don't forget to share with them your goals and motivations for following this diet. There will be days when intermittent fasting will be a breeze, whereas others will feel like an uphill battle. On days like these, your support system will grant you the motivation you need to keep going. If possible, find a dieting buddy. When you have someone else going through the same, the chances of sticking to the diet will increase. Also, it becomes fun. Today, several online support groups and chat rooms are available as well. You can use these platforms to connect with others who are following similar dietary protocols. Exchanging tips and sharing your experiences can help you push through and make you feel better and more confident about the diet.

Prioritize Protein Intake

Regardless of what you wish to eat or not, be sure to consume plenty of protein and complex carbs. These two food categories promote satiety and provide your body with all the nutrients needed. They are also relatively low in calories. There will be days when you feel like breaking the fast earlier or binging on something unhealthy. On days like these, consume all the required macros and essential nutrients before reaching for something sweet. This also reduces the risk of overeating. Fill yourself up with lean meat, lentils, legumes, healthy vegetables, and other forms of protein before succumbing to junk food. Once your hunger is satiated, the craving will automatically fade away.

Alternatively, you can also follow the delayed gratification technique to ensure that you don't give in to your cravings. The idea is quite simple: whenever a craving strikes you, take a break, breathe deeply, slowly sip on a glass of water, and make a note of your craving. Maintain a list of different foods you want to eat. Whenever you want to eat something, write it down. This simple act of expressing what you desire takes away some of the power the craving has over you. This also increases the chances of following a diet without any slip-ups.

Whenever you eat, make sure that you do not skimp on portion size. Remember, your body needs sufficient calories to function efficiently and effectively. If you starve yourself while fasting all day long, it does not promote weight loss. Instead, you will just end up doing more harm than good.

Plan to Deal with Hunger Pangs

One of the most common culprits for why people tend to give up on diets is hunger. Hunger pangs can quickly derail even the most motivated dieters. You should not only expect hunger pangs but prepare for them, too. You can tackle these spurs of hunger by adding calorie-free beverages, consuming more whole foods and satiating meals, or practicing delayed gratification. Perhaps the simplest one is to keep yourself busy. After all, if your brain is thoroughly engaged, whether it's working, reading, or enjoying music, you won't get a chance to think about your next meal.

Following the simple and practical advice in this chapter, jumping on the intermittent fasting bandwagon will be easier than ever.

Chapter 8: How to Keep Motivated While Fasting

It goes without saying that motivation is important in every aspect of life. The one difference between those who succeed and those trying to "make it" is their motivation. Internal motivation grants you the energy and reasons to keep going despite all obstacles and hurdles. In this section, let's look at a couple of simple tips you can follow to keep yourself motivated while following intermittent fasting.

Make a List of Your Goals

Goals give you a sense of purpose and direction. Without goals, chances are you will never get anywhere you want to be. Whether it's your personal or professional life, goals are necessary, and dieting is no exception. Now, before you start dieting, you need to understand your reasons for doing so. If you have no reason, what is the point of making all these changes? Make a list of all the different goals you want to achieve; be it weight loss and regulation or improving your overall state of health. You can have multiple goals. Once you have a few goals, list them in order of priority.

While setting goals, make sure they are SMART: Small, Measurable, Attainable, Relevant, and Time-bound. Unless all these elements are present, the chances of accomplishing those goals are reduced. Not setting goals is as dangerous as setting vague ones. For instance, a vague goal would be, "I want to lose weight." Instead, a good and clearly defined goal is, "I want to lose fifteen pounds within four months." This goal is doable and realistic. It also has a time limit, which will lower the chances of procrastination creeping in.

Have an Accountability Partner

It is a natural human tendency to behave or act according to what you say. Before you start the diet, talk to your support team about the diet and why you're following it. In a way, you are creating an external source of accountability. Now that you have shared your dreams and goals with someone else, the pressure to achieve those goals and to prove yourself become quite high. This is where accountability comes into play. Yes, you are personally accountable for yourself and your achievements, but external accountability works better.

If possible, find an accountability partner. Keeping track of your progress and sharing it with one person daily can be a positive and motivating experience. Enlisting a friend or an accountability buddy while you are getting started on this new journey will increase your likelihood of success. In today's world, we are all connected through the Internet, so regardless of where your accountability buddy is, you can always reach them with ease. If you want, you can also join an online community to that end.

Establish Short-Term Goals

We just mentioned that you need to establish certain goals for yourself while dieting. Now, it is time to establish a few short-term goals. Remember that any long-term objective can be easily broken down into multiple short-term goals. It's easier to achieve short-term goals, and every success that comes your way increases your motivation to keep going. After all, a long-term goal is nothing more than a combination and amalgamation of several short-term milestones. For instance, if you want to lose 15 lbs in four months, this can be further broken down into short-term goals. Like, "Following the intermittent fasting protocol for seven days straight" or "Exercising daily for thirty minutes." By breaking down the long-term objective into short-term goals, achieving the goal seems more realistic, practical, and achievable.

It isn't just important to establish goals but to decide on the rewards for attaining them, too. Why achieve a goal if there is no reward down the line? The rewards can be anything you want, except food! If the reward is food-related, it will soon undo all the benefits of fasting. Instead, it could be something like treating yourself to a manicure, buying those clothes you have meant to, or going out for a long drive. Whatever the activity is, make sure that you treat yourself to it after achieving each of your short-term goals.

Inspiring Content

The human brain is incredibly powerful, and you need to be mindful of all that you feed it. In our modern, ultra-connected world, we are constantly surrounded by information. If you don't start filtering what you're feeding your brain, it will quickly be overwhelmed. Your brain regulates your level of motivation. The simplest way to make sure you are highly motivated while following this diet is by feeding it motivational content. There is no need to do this for hours and hours; even ten minutes dedicated to feeding your brain quality inspirational content can do wonders. From watching YouTube videos and listening to podcasts to reading, there are many options available.

At times, especially when making a dietary change, it might not be easy, and you might feel all alone in your journey. These thoughts can quickly derail you and prevent you from fasting. As a guiding principle, no one is truly alone unless they believe it; others will always experience similar situations. So, dedicate a little time to read about others and their journeys, struggles, and successes.

Alternatively, turn your goals into positive affirmations and repeat them daily for five minutes, like a mantra. This is a simple exercise that can boost your motivation. Start your day with a couple of positive affirmations, and your motivation levels will stay high.

The Carrot and the Stick

Even the rewards may not seem that tempting or enticing enough to follow a diet. What can you do in these situations? Now, it's time for the carrot and the stick approach. This is a very simple technique, thanks to the analogy it uses. According to this technique, to motivate a donkey to move further along, you can either motivate it with a carrot or strike it with a stick. It implies motivation through reward or punishment. Punishment doesn't mean physically punishing yourself; it could be a sense of deprivation that acts as punishment. For instance, reward yourself with a spa day if you follow the diet for a whole month. Now, what would be the punishment if you do not achieve this goal? Perhaps you can eliminate one of your favorite foods from your diet for a couple of weeks. Or maybe increase the time spent working out. The idea of having to do something you don't want to can push you further and motivate you to do better.

Creative Visualization

Forget about establishing rewards or punishments for motivating yourself for a moment. Instead, there is another simple technique you can use, known as positive visualizations. In this technique, you close your eyes and picture a specific outcome or a scenario in your mind's eye. Visualization triggers your imagination, creativity, and jogs your memories. In parallel, it can tingle all your senses and awaken you from the inside. The next time you are running low on motivation, close your eyes and take a break from whatever you are doing for five minutes. Visualize how your life will be once you have attained your goals. How will you feel once you are fitter, healthier, or at your ideal body weight? How do you feel about yourself? How does life feel? Thinking about these questions and answering them honestly will provide several reasons why following the diet is desirable and the "right thing to do." This also gives you the instant motivation to keep going.

While using visualization, you can also use it to contemplate whether you are on the right path. For instance, close your eyes, and visualize how your life will be in the next six or twelve months if you quit the diet right now. It helps you take stock of your life and concentrate on making healthy and desirable changes voluntarily. If you are not willing to make these changes, following the diet will quickly become unbearable in the long run. Unless it comes from within, no one else can compel or force you.

Set fifteen minutes aside to reflect on your goals and where you want to be in life. You can also use positive affirmations that are meaningful to you and practice them daily. Managing your motivation levels is not difficult, provided you are interested and invested in doing so.

Focus on the Positives

Apart from visualizing a bright and healthy future, concentrate on the immediate positive aspects of fasting. This diet is bound to make you feel more confident, energetic, and productive. Whenever you attain a small goal, your motivation levels will increase. If you have never followed a diet before, imagine how you will feel if you follow intermittent fasting for ten days. If you have never exercised for a day in your life before, imagine the happiness of realizing that you have completed two weeks at the gym. These are the small positives associated with intermittent fasting. All it takes is a little time and commitment from you to see all the wonderful results it offers.

Focus on each of the positive feelings you experience daily while following this diet. It can be something as simple as saying no to dessert after eating or not adding sugar to your morning cup of coffee. You might not consciously think about these things or believe they are significant achievements, but they are. Every little positive step you take matters immensely. By celebrating them, your motivation and commitment will go through the roof.

Be Compassionate

You need to be compassionate, not just to others, but toward yourself as well. There will be days when you don't feel motivated, and it feels like an uphill battle. You probably realize the week or month ahead will not go according to what you might have planned. Instead of indulging in pointless negative talk, it's time to become mindful of your inner critic. Engaging in self-criticism and negative self-talk is quite easy, but this won't take you far.

On the contrary, finding something positive to concentrate on is seldom easy. If you want to attain your long-term objectives, it is important to tame your inner critic. Rather than focus solely on everything that isn't going right, concentrate on the good.

Apart from this, turn all the negative talk into positive self-talk. If you feel demotivated that you cannot get through the fasting window, tell yourself you possess the inner strength to complete the fast. By showing a little compassion toward yourself and being aware of your own strengths and weaknesses, your motivation levels will also increase.

Check Your Progress

Lastly, one important thing you need to do is continually check the progress you make. Even if it is just a week, there will be progress. Whether it is a slight fluctuation in your body weight or a general feeling of improvement in your life, there are different ways to check your progress. You will learn more about all this in the next chapter. For now, it is crucial to understand that motivation is something that is well within your control. No one else can motivate you unless you find that spark within. Another great thing about motivation is it increases your self-awareness.

Chapter 9: Non-Scale Victories and Fasting Setbacks

We just mentioned how important it is to measure the progress you make while fasting. Measuring progress is vital in order to understand the distance you've covered in life. Victories are not always measurable, and wins such as getting through a fasting day without thinking of giving up are also progress. Generally speaking, you cannot achieve success without failure. You will inevitably run into obstacles. You should not only expect this but must prepare yourself for it as well. When you are prepared, dealing with any potential setbacks becomes more manageable. In this chapter, you will learn about certain "non-scale victories" you should pay attention to and how to deal with setbacks throughout your intermittent fasting journey.

Non-Scale Victories to Celebrate

Whether you want to lose weight or lead a healthier life, none of this is going to be an overnight journey. It is a multifaceted process that requires sustained commitment and the development of healthier and more desirable habits. Non-scale victories, or NSVs, are simple health improvements resulting from small changes to your daily lifestyle. If the scale is your measure of success, you will forget all the small victories that come every step of the way. It is rather unfair that your journey to a healthier life and its efforts are reduced to a mere number on a scale. The number on the scale does not and cannot reflect all the changes you have made in your daily life. In this section, let us look at some simple non-scale victories most people forget to celebrate.

While following the 16/8 intermittent fasting protocol, chances are you will start feeling more energetic than you ever did. You are essentially consuming a healthy diet, exercising regularly, and getting sufficient sleep. Combining all these factors makes it abundantly clear how a simple diet can make you feel more energetic. By feeding your body all the nutrients and physical activity it needs to function effectively, its overall productivity and efficiency is guaranteed to improve.

Perhaps the most important non-scale victory you need to pay attention to is how your clothes fit. Even if there is no dip or fluctuation in your weight on the scale, chances are your clothes will fit you better after two weeks of intermittent fasting. At times, weight loss isn't always visible. This is especially true for fat loss. When your clothes fit better, you can see that this diet is working and delivering the expected results. According to the research conducted by Courtney Maclin-Akinyemi et al. (2017), among 77% of women and over 35% of men who wanted to lose weight, their clothes fitted them better. So, start paying attention to how your clothes fit as you advance through the fasting protocol.

If you have successfully shifted to an intermittent fasting lifestyle, chances are your sleep pattern has also improved. When you have a proper schedule in place and are sticking to it, it becomes easier to tire your body and brain out at the end of the day. For instance, exercising regularly is believed to regulate your internal sleep cycle. Even losing body fat has a positive effect on sleep and its quality.

According to the research conducted by Soohyun Nam et al. (2018), weight loss can improve your quality of sleep over time.

It isn't secret knowledge that exercise has multiple health benefits. If you exercise more than you ever did, your fitness will improve, and you might not have even noticed it yet. Slowly, you will notice that you can exercise for longer, perform more reps, and even lift heavier weights. All these changes are an indication that you are progressing in the right direction. When the intensity and duration of exercise increases gradually, it shows you that your body has come a long way. This is a fitness milestone that you have attained—do not forget to celebrate it.

According to a study by Nicola Veronese et al. (2017), weight loss can improve your memory, increase your attention span, and support quicker mental processing. This goes to show that any improvement in your physical health will assist your cognitive functioning, too.

A wonderful thing about intermittent fasting is it promotes the concept of healthy and wholesome eating instead of mindlessly bingeing on processed foods. By eliminating all undesirable food from your diet, such as those rich in trans fats and unhealthy sugars, and by replacing them with healthier fruit, vegetables, and wholesome ingredients, there will be a positive effect. According to the study conducted by Rajani Katta et al. (2014), your skin's health can improve when you limit dairy products and high glycemic index foods. Since intermittent fasting encourages the consumption of fruit and vegetables rich in antioxidants and a variety of nutrients and vitamins, this will promote visibly clearer and smoother skin over time.

Perhaps the most important non-scale victory you need to celebrate is when you have lost inches. If you are exercising daily by engaging in weight or strength training, your body measurements will change. As such, one of the most important numbers you need to keep track of is your waist circumference. Before you start this diet, measure yourself and make a list of your body measurements. Also, monitor your waist to hip ratio. All the healthy, desirable lifestyle habits and changes (and sacrifices) you are making now will certainly pay off.

Let's not forget that your emotional state affects your eating patterns. If you take a moment and think about it, this makes perfect sense. Chances are you feel like eating something sweet when you're feeling sad, something crunchy when you're upset, or junk food when you're bored. This is because of dopamine released in the brain, a chemical associated with the "feel-good" or reward feeling. Stress eating is also referred to as emotional eating, and it activates the "eat and reward" connection in your brain. If you no longer reach for food to cope with any stress you are experiencing, it is an important victory that you cannot ignore.

As you start losing weight, the stress on your muscles and joints will diminish. This is especially true for the weight-bearing ones in your back and legs. With weight loss, your joint pain will also be reduced. This, in turn, makes it easier to become more physically active and fit, which will promote further weight loss.

One healthy lifestyle change that intermittent fasting will introduce you to is home cooking. Cooking at home can be incredibly fun and exciting once you start following the different recipes provided in this book. It also gives you better control over your body's nutritional requirements and the cooking process. Combined, these factors are bound to improve your relationship with food. Another notable benefit of cooking at home regularly is that it will lighten your financial expenses. If you are used to ordering take-out or other convenience foods, you have probably been spending a lot more than you realized. Your bank balance will certainly thank you once you start cooking at home! You can also set aside a monthly food budget to accommodate all your dietary needs and requirements without any hassle.

Another non-scale victory is an improvement in your overall mood. When you start eating better, exercising regularly, and sleeping through the night like a baby, your mood will automatically improve. As mentioned earlier, if you have recognized any emotional eating patterns and managed to hit a breakthrough, you can now handle stress without reaching for food. Combining all these essential elements will automatically make you feel better about yourself and everything you undertake. When your mood is better, your overall performance and productivity will also skyrocket.

In parallel, you need to regularly check certain health markers such as blood sugar and blood pressure. In the previous chapter, you were introduced to the various benefits of intermittent fasting and scientific evidence that backs these claims. If you regularly follow the protocol, do not forget to check your blood sugar and blood pressure levels. If you notice an improvement in both of these health markers, it means the diet is working for you.

Losing weight can be a health goal in itself. Measuring weight loss from time to time is perfectly normal. Still, as established, this is not the only means to determine your success while dieting. Most of the non-scale victories discussed in this section may not reflect in your weight, but they're worth celebrating. With every little win that comes your way, your motivation for following this diet will increase. When you know you are making healthy changes and they are paying off, you will feel better.

Fasting Setbacks to Tackle

You can lose weight and keep it off with intermittent fasting. This is perhaps the most common reason why people turn to this diet. By fasting for sixteen hours, your body's metabolism increases and accelerates weight loss. You may be wondering what the common weight loss benefit offered by this diet is. Diets take time to show results. This stands true for intermittent fasting, too. As long as you follow this diet for at least eight to ten weeks, you will witness positive changes. During this period, you can expect to lose anywhere between 6-10 lbs. The journey of weight loss is not an overnight process; you did not gain all those excess pounds overnight, so how can you lose them immediately? Different factors come into play when it comes to weight loss. Your gender, level of activity, and dietary choices will command your weight loss journey.

Do not compare your weight loss results with someone else and feel bad (remember, no negative self-perception!). Realize that the results will vary from one person to another. If you are not losing weight, chances are something isn't right in your diet planning or execution. In this upcoming section, let's look at some fasting setbacks and how you can tackle them efficiently.

Eating Too Much after Fasting

Perhaps the most common mistake many people make when they start fasting is that they overeat once their eating window starts. Don't think of the eating window as the timeframe to compensate for the fasting period. If weight loss is your priority, your calorie expenditure needs to exceed your calorie intake. If you consume more calories during the eating window than before intermittent fasting, you won't notice any weight loss. If all the calories you normally consume were shifted to the eating period, this diet would not make any sense.

Instead of eating too much, eat until you are full. To do this, adopt the habit of eating slowly, chewing thoroughly, and making healthier dietary choices. Putting your fork down between each bite can also help if you're a fast eater. Unless you do all this, you cannot see positive change. If you want, you can also use a calorie counting app during the initial days to make healthier choices. No, you don't have to count every calorie you ingest, but becoming aware of what you eat will help with weight loss.

Not Eating Nutritious Food

We've established and reiterated that intermittent fasting protocols are more about when you eat than what you eat. Intermittent fasting should not become your excuse for eating whatever you want during the eating window. If weight loss is your goal, consuming calorie-dense foods such as prepackaged and processed junk food will not promote weight loss (quite the opposite). Instead, your primary focus should be nutrient-dense foods. You were introduced to various foods you can safely consume during intermittent fasting in the previous section. Fill up on healthy fats, lean protein, and fiber-rich carbohydrates to reduce your overall calorie intake and promote satiety. It doesn't mean you need to deprive yourself of the foods you love and enjoy. As long as treats like chocolate and ice cream are occasional and within reasonable limits, you don't have to deprive yourself of anything.

Skipping Meals during the Eating Window

If you don't eat sufficient food during the eating window, sustaining your body through fasting quickly becomes difficult. If you starve yourself pointlessly by skipping meals, it increases hunger pangs, making it more difficult to stick to your schedule. Restricting yourself too much also increases the risk of overeating or bingeing on unhealthy foods when your fasting window ends. Apart from all this, you are depriving your body of the essential nutrients it requires. Remember, it was mentioned that shifting to starvation mode is never ideal. Once your body is in the starvation stage, it stops burning calories and instead starts protecting and harboring them. This can result in weight gain rather than weight loss.

Do not overindulge during the eating window. Instead, you need to eat until your hunger is satisfied. Doing a little meal prep on the weekends makes it easier to prepare the required meals during the week since most of the work is already done. When you know a meal is ready and waiting for you, the chances of getting thrown off schedule are dramatically reduced.

Not Fasting Long Enough

There will be days when it feels like you cannot complete the entire sixteen hours of fasting. On days like these, listen to your body, but don't make a habit of it. You need to fast for sixteen hours if you want to see the positive results promised by this diet. If you regularly skip fasting, what good is trying in the first place? If you want to reap the benefits of this diet, you need to fast for at least fourteen hours daily. By following the schedule, you slowly get your body accustomed to eating during a specific window and fasting for the rest of the day. After that, all that is required is commitment and self-control.

You Are Not Sleeping Properly

The importance of sleep should never be overlooked when it comes to improving and maintaining your overall health and wellbeing. Sleep not only awards your body the rest it needs, but it affects your metabolism. Improper sleep increases certain hunger-inducing hormones, which makes it difficult to stick to the fasting schedule. Also, when you sleep, your body finally gets a chance to work on actively digesting whatever you have consumed during the eating window. Make an effort to sleep for at least seven to eight hours daily. It is not just the duration of the sleep that matters; quality is just as important. You need to get good quality sleep every night, which can be promoted by a warm shower and aromatherapy.

Not Drinking Enough Water

Drinking plenty of water and staying hydrated can never be underestimated. This point has been repeatedly stressed in this book because dehydration is quite common, and many people forget about it. Another important benefit of drinking sufficient water is that it quells hunger. At times, you may feel hungry, only to realize that a big cup of water is all you needed.

Exercising Too Much

It can be quite tempting to exercise more vigorously and for longer while shifting to this diet. After all, exercising is important for weight loss and maintenance in general. Unfortunately, it doesn't help—at least initially—so don't go overboard and don't push your body beyond its limits. Exercising too hard and not eating enough is a recipe for disaster. Instead of attaining your weight loss goals, it will harm your body and health in the long run. Over-exercising or working out more intensively than required while reducing food intake will augment your hunger and reduce your energy levels. As a result, you may also overeat and binge on unhealthy calories. During the initial couple of days, make sure your exercise routine is quite light. Once your body is accustomed to fasting, you can gradually increase the intensity of your workout routine. Remember, this is a long-term plan and not an overnight process.

Lack of Planning

One of the most common mistakes people make while shifting to intermittent fasting is that they don't plan. You need to plan, and there is no way around it. As we've seen, coming up with an intermittent fasting schedule is not a Herculean task. Once you target your lifestyle needs and requirements, simply adjust them according to this diet. If you keep cutting corners or cheating on your meal plan from one week to another, the yields will not be worth the effort you exert. Consistency is fundamental because intermittent fasting is more of a lifestyle than just another diet. Plan all your meals and snacks. Prepare a few snacks and meals and keep them handy. Also, don't forget to stock your pantry with the required nutrient-dense ingredients. This makes following the diet a breeze. It also gives you enough flexibility to decide what you want to eat and switch things up from time to time.

Feeling Guilty

Be patient and consistent in your efforts while shifting to intermittent fasting. There will be days when you need to break your fast ahead of schedule, or ones when you cannot fast at all. If you want to follow this diet, make it sustainable, and uphold your commitment, then you should not feel guilty or ashamed when you cannot complete the fast. These negative feelings can prevent you from getting back on track the following day. There will be setbacks, inevitably, but it's best to focus on your commitment. It is okay if you cannot complete your fast one day. As long as you start fasting the next day, you have nothing to worry about. Cut yourself some slack, and don't take these setbacks personally. Instead, concentrate on your journey and all the progress you are making.

At the end of the day, progress is impossible without setbacks. So, don't get discouraged, and instead, follow the simple steps and suggestions given in this chapter to make things easier.

Chapter 10: Intermittent Fasting 16/8 Recipes and Meal Plan

Meal Shakes

Peanut Butter Cup Shake

Number of servings: 2

Nutritional values per serving:

Calories – 260

Fat – 6 grams

Carbohydrates – 21 grams

Protein – 30 grams

Ingredients:

- 1 cup unsweetened almond milk
- 2 tablespoons cocoa powder
- 1 tablespoon natural peanut butter
- 2 scoops vanilla or chocolate plant-based protein powder
- 1 frozen banana, sliced
- Water, as required (optional)

Directions:

1. Pour almond milk into the blender. Add cocoa, peanut butter, protein powder, and banana.

2. Blend until you get a smooth puree.

3. If the shake looks too thick, add water and blend until smooth. You can add ice as well.

4. Pour into two tall glasses and serve.

Dark Chocolate Peppermint Shake

Number of servings: 2

Nutritional values per serving:

Calories – 295

Fat – 6 grams

Carbohydrates – 49 grams

Protein – 22 grams

Ingredients:

- 2 large frozen bananas, sliced
- 2 cups non-dairy milk of your preference
- 4 tablespoons cocoa powder
- 2 tablespoons dark chocolate chips (optional)
- 2 scoops of whey chocolate protein powder
- ½ teaspoon pure peppermint extract
- Ice cubes, as required
- 1/8 teaspoon salt

Directions:

1. Place banana, cocoa, protein powder, salt, and peppermint extract into the blender.
2. Pour milk and blend the mixture until nice and smooth. Add dark chocolate chips if you are using them and blend until smooth.
3. Add ice cubes and blend once again.
4. Enjoy the shake in tall glasses.

Strawberry Cheesecake Shake

Number of servings: 2

Nutritional values per serving:

Calories – 210

Fat – 5 grams

Carbohydrates – 7 grams

Protein – 30 grams

Ingredients:

- 2 cups almond milk
- 2/3 cup whey protein powder
- 1 cup frozen strawberries
- 2 tablespoons light cream cheese

Directions:

1. Pour almond milk into the blender. Add protein powder, strawberries, and cream cheese.

2. Blend for few seconds until you get a smooth puree.

3. Pour into two tall glasses and serve.

Very Berry Super Shake

Number of servings: 1

Nutritional values per serving:

Calories – 500

Fat – 11 grams

Carbohydrates – 54 grams

Protein – 57 grams

Ingredients:

- ¾ cup water
- 1 cup frozen mixed berries
- 1 scoop vanilla protein powder
- ½ tablespoon ground flaxseeds
- ½ cup spinach
- ¼ cup plain, low-fat yogurt
- ½ tablespoon walnuts

Directions:

1. Place berries, water, vanilla protein powder, flaxseeds, spinach, yogurt, and walnuts into a blender.

2. Blend the mixture until you get a smooth puree.

3. Pour into a tall glass and serve.

Pineapple Green Smoothie

Number of servings: 2

Nutritional values per serving:

Calories – 295

Fat – 5.5 grams

Carbohydrates – 54 grams

Protein – 13 grams

Ingredients:

- 1 cup unsweetened almond milk
- 2 cups baby spinach
- 1 cup frozen pineapple chunks
- 2 – 7 teaspoons pure maple syrup or honey (optional)
- 2/3 cup nonfat, plain Greek yogurt
- 2 medium frozen bananas, sliced
- 2 tablespoons chia seeds

Directions:

1. Pour yogurt and almond milk into the blender. Place spinach, chia seeds, pineapple, banana, and maple syrup into the blender.

2. Keep blending until you get a smooth puree.

3. Pour into two tall glasses and serve.

Strawberry Chocolate Smoothie

Number of servings: 2

Nutritional values per serving:

Calories – 305

Fat – 13.4 grams

Carbohydrates – 46.8 grams

Protein – 7.4 grams

Ingredients:

- 3 cups frozen strawberries
- 2 tablespoons almond butter
- 2 tablespoons honey
- 2 cups chilled, unsweetened, chocolate almond milk
- 2 tablespoons unsweetened cocoa powder

Directions:

1. Place strawberries and cocoa powder into the blender. Add honey and milk. Then add the almond butter.

2. Blend until nice and smooth. Once smooth, pour into two glasses and serve.

Carrot Apple Smoothie

Number of servings: 1

Nutritional values per serving:

Calories – 245

Fat – 8 grams

Carbohydrates – 46 grams

Protein – 4 grams

Ingredients:

- 1 large carrot, sliced
- ½ large honey crisp apple, cored, cut in two
- 1 tablespoon fresh lemon juice
- 1 teaspoon minced fresh turmeric or ½ teaspoon turmeric powder
- ½ medium ripe banana, sliced
- ½ cup light coconut milk
- 1 teaspoon minced fresh ginger
- Ice cubes, as required

Directions:

1. Pour coconut milk into the blender. Add ginger, carrot, turmeric, apple, lemon juice, and banana.

2. Blitz until you get a smooth puree. Now add the ice cubes and blend.

3. Pour into a tall glass and serve.

Mango Raspberry Smoothie

Number of servings: 2

Nutritional values per serving:

Calories – 190

Fat – 7.4 grams

Carbohydrates – 32 grams

Protein – 1.5 grams

Ingredients:

- 1 cup water
- 2 tablespoons lemon juice
- ½ cup frozen raspberries
- ½ medium avocado, peeled, pitted, chopped
- 1 ½ cups frozen mango
- 2 tablespoons agave nectar

Directions:

1. Place avocado, mango, lemon juice, agave nectar, and raspberries into a blender. Pour water and blitz until you get a smooth puree.

2. Pour into two tall glasses and serve with crushed ice if desired.

Strawberry Oat Smoothie

Number of servings: 2

Nutritional values per serving:

Calories - 280

Fat - 2 grams

Carbohydrates - 56 grams

Protein - 13 grams

Ingredients:

- 2 cups sliced strawberries
- 2 cups nonfat milk
- 2 teaspoons honey
- Ice cubes, as required
- 1 banana, sliced
- ½ cup rolled oats
- ½ teaspoon vanilla extract

Directions:

1. Place oats, strawberries, honey, ice cubes, vanilla, and banana into a blender.

2. Pour milk on top and blitz until you get a smooth puree.

3. Pour into two tall glasses and serve.

Raspberry Peanut Butter Smoothie

Number of servings: 2

Nutritional values per serving:

Calories – 270

Fat – 12 grams

Carbohydrates – 38 grams

Protein – 7 grams

Ingredients:

- 1 banana, sliced
- 2 cups almond milk
- 1 cup ice as required
- 2 cups raspberries
- 2 tablespoons peanut butter

Directions:

1. Place banana, almond milk, ice, raspberries, and peanut butter into the blender.
2. Blend until you get a smooth puree.
3. Pour into two glasses and serve.

Flax Seed Smoothie

Number of servings: 2

Nutritional values per serving:

Calories – 275

Fat – 8 grams

Carbohydrates – 47 grams

Protein – 7.5 grams

Ingredients:

- 1 frozen banana, sliced
- 4 tablespoons flaxseed meal
- 2 cups frozen strawberries
- 2 cups low-fat vanilla soymilk

Directions:

1. Place strawberries, banana slices, and flaxseed meal into a blender.

2. Pour soymilk on top. Blitz until you get a smooth puree.

3. Pour into two tall glasses. Serve with crushed ice if desired.

Breakfast Recipes

Veggie Mini Quiches

Number of servings: 3

Nutritional values per serving: (4 mini quiches)

Calories – 95

Fat – 6.8 grams

Carbohydrates – 2 grams

Protein – 6 grams

Ingredients:

- 1 teaspoon coconut oil
- 1 medium carrot, grated
- 2 large eggs, whisked
- Salt to taste
- 1/3heaped cup zucchini
- 1 green onion, finely chopped (keep the greens and whites separate)
- 3 tablespoons grated Monterrey Jack cheese

Directions:

1. Take a mini cupcake pan and spray cooking spray into the wells. You need to spray oil into 12 of the wells.

2. Take a skillet and keep it over medium flame. Pour oil into the skillet and let it heat.

3. Once the oil is heated, add whites of the green onion, carrots, and zucchini and stir-fry for a few minutes until the vegetables are soft. Turn off the heat and stir in the greens of the green onion. Let cool completely.

4. Crack the eggs into a bowl and beat well. Add the sautéed vegetables, salt, and cheese and stir.

5. Pour the egg mixture into the prepared muffin pan.

6. Bake the mini quiches in an oven that has been preheated to 350°F, for about 15-18 minutes or until the eggs are set.

7. Let the mini quiches cool in the pan for 15 minutes. Take a knife and run it around the edges of the quiches to loosen them from the mold.

8. The mini quiches are ready to serve now.

Ham, Egg, and Avocado Breakfast Burrito

Number of servings: 4

Nutritional values per serving:

Calories – 400

Fat – 24 grams

Carbohydrates – 36 grams

Protein – 16 grams

Ingredients:

- 4 eggs
- 1 cup cooked, diced ham
- 4 large whole wheat tortillas
- 2 tablespoons milk
- 2 avocadoes, peeled, pitted, sliced
- Grated cheese

Directions:

1. Beat eggs in a microwave-safe greased bowl. Add milk and whisk well.

2. Place the bowl in the microwave and cook on high for about a minute. Stir the eggs and place them back in the microwave. Continue cooking until the eggs are set.

3. Make four equal portions of the eggs, avocado, ham, and cheese. Scatter one portion of each, along the diameter of each of the tortillas.

4. Wrap the tortillas like a burrito. The burritos are ready to serve.

5. If desired, you can also cook the burritos in a skillet or a Panini press until golden brown. The choice is yours.

Cauliflower English Muffins

Number of servings: 8

Nutritional values per serving: (2 muffins per serving, without toppings)

Calories – 170

Fat – 11 grams

Carbohydrates – 7.5 grams

Protein – 10.5 grams

Ingredients:

- 10 cups cauliflower florets (around 2 pounds)
- 2 large eggs, lightly beaten
- 2 cups sharp cheddar cheese
- ¼ teaspoon salt

Directions:

1. Take two large baking trays and place a sheet of parchment paper on each.

2. Process the cauliflower in the food processor until you get a rice-like texture.

3. Place the cauliflower rice in a microwave-safe bowl. Cover the bowl loosely and cook the cauliflower on High in a microwave for 4 minutes.

4. Take a large piece of kitchen cloth. Place cauliflower on the center of the cloth. Bring the edges of the cloth together and squeeze the cauliflower to remove extra moisture.

5. Place the squeezed cauliflower in a bowl along with eggs, cheddar cheese, and salt and mix until well combined.

6. Take a 3-inch biscuit cutter and place it on one corner of the baking sheet. Place about ¼ cup of the cauliflower mixture inside the cutter. Press lightly and carefully remove the biscuit cutter.

7. Leave a one-inch gap and repeat this process. When the baking sheet is full, place the cauliflower similarly on the other baking sheet. You should have 16 muffins in total.

8. Place the baking tray in an oven that has been preheated to 425°F for about 25-30 minutes or until you can see them browning around the edges.

9. You can use your own favorite toppings to serve the muffins. You can use them to make sandwiches as well.

Broccoli and Parmesan Cheese Omelet

Number of servings: 2

Nutritional values per serving: (1 omelet)

Calories – 410

Fat – 20 grams

Carbohydrates – 22 grams

Protein – 33 grams

Ingredients:

- 4 large egg whites
- 4 large eggs
- 2 teaspoons extra-virgin olive oil
- 2 shallots, finely chopped
- 2 slices sprouted grain bread
- 1 cup chopped broccoli
- ½ cup finely grated parmesan cheese

Directions:

1. Place eggs and egg whites in a bowl and whisk well.

2. Pour oil into a small skillet and heat over medium flame. Once the oil is heated, add shallots and broccoli and cook until the broccoli turns bright green.

3. Remove half the broccoli mixture from the pan and place it in a bowl.

4. Spread the remaining broccoli mixture all over the skillet.

5. Pour half the egg mixture into the pan, all over the broccoli, making sure not to stir.

6. Scatter half the cheese on top. Cook covered until the eggs are cooked. Remove omelet onto a plate.

7. Make the other omelet using the broccoli mixture that was set aside, the remaining cheese, and the remaining egg mixture.

8. Meanwhile, toast the bread slices the desired amount.

9. To assemble: place a slice of toast on individual serving plates.

10. Place an omelet on each piece of toast and serve. You can fold the omelet in half or a quarter before placing it on the toast.

Summer Skillet Vegetable and Egg Scramble

Number of servings: 2

Nutritional values per serving: (1-½ cups portion)

Calories – 255

Fat – 14 grams

Carbohydrates – 19.5 grams

Protein – 12.5 grams

Ingredients:

- 1 tablespoon olive oil
- 2 cups thinly sliced mixed vegetables (mushroom, zucchini, and bell pepper)
- ½ teaspoon minced fresh herbs of your choice
- 1 cup packed baby kale or baby spinach
- 6 ounces baby potatoes, thinly sliced
- 1 ½ scallions, thinly sliced (keep the greens and whites separate)
- 3 large eggs, lightly beaten
- ¼ teaspoon salt or to taste

Directions:

1. Pour oil into a large skillet and heat over medium flame. When the oil is heated, add potatoes and stir.

2. Keep the skillet covered and cook until slightly soft. Make sure you stir often.

3. Stir in mixed vegetables and whites of the scallions and cook until vegetables are light brown and slightly soft.

4. Add the fresh herbs and stir. Push the vegetables to the edges of the skillet.

5. Lower the heat to medium-low. Place scallion greens in the center of the skillet. Add eggs over the scallion greens and stir. Cook until the eggs are soft-cooked, stirring often.

6. Add kale into the egg mixture and stir. Turn off the heat.

7. Now mix the egg scramble and the vegetables. Add salt and stir.

8. Divide onto two plates and serve.

Loaded Baked Potato Breakfast Casserole

Number of servings: 4

Nutritional values per serving:

Calories – 165

Fat – 10 grams

Carbohydrates – 8 grams

Protein – 11 grams

Ingredients:

- 6 ounces baby potatoes
- ¼ cup light sour cream + extra for serving
- ¼ cup milk
- ½ cup chopped green bell pepper
- 2 thick slices bacon, cooked, crumbled + extra for serving
- 4 eggs
- ½ teaspoon salt
- ¼ cup shredded cheddar cheese + extra for serving
- 1 green onion, sliced + extra for serving
- Pepper to taste

Directions:

1. Prepare a baking sheet by lining it with aluminum foil. Place potatoes on the baking sheet.

2. Place the baking sheet in an oven that has been preheated to 400°F and bake for about 30 minutes or until the potatoes are cooked.

3. Take out the baking sheet from the oven and let the potatoes cool. Chop the potatoes into smaller pieces.

4. Now, set the oven temperature to 350°F and wait for the temperature to reduce.

5. Take a baking dish of about 6 – 7 inches or use a small casserole dish and grease it with cooking spray.

6. Beat the eggs in a bowl while adding milk, sour cream, and salt. Add potatoes, bacon, onion, bell pepper, and cheese and stir until well incorporated.

7. Transfer the mixture into the baking dish and place the dish in the oven.

8. Set the timer for about 30 minutes and let it bake until the eggs are cooked in the middle. If you see the edges are getting brown and the center is not cooked, cover the dish with foil and bake.

9. Garnish with green onion, bacon, and cheese. Drizzle sour cream on top and serve.

Layered Chia Pudding with Mixed Fruit Puree

Number of servings: 4

Nutritional values per serving: (1 glass)

Calories – 685

Fat – 35 grams

Carbohydrates – 74 grams

Protein – 24 grams

Ingredients:

For chia pudding:

- 1 cup chia seeds
- 2 teaspoons vanilla extract
- 4 cups almond milk or any other plant-based milk of your choice
- 2 tablespoons maple syrup

For parfait:

- 2 large mangoes, peeled, cubed
- 2 cups raspberries
- 4 kiwis, peeled, cubed
- 4 tablespoons yogurt or coconut yogurt or soy yogurt
- 4 tablespoons hemp hearts

Directions:

1. Combine almond milk, maple syrup, and vanilla extract in a bowl.

2. Stir in the chia seeds. Keep stirring for a couple of minutes.

3. Cover the bowl and keep the bowl in the refrigerator for about an hour or until thick.

4. While the pudding is chilling, prepare the fruit puree. For this, blend the kiwis in a blender. Once you get a smooth puree, pour it into a bowl.

5. Rinse the blender and now place mangoes into the blender. Blend the mangoes until you get a smooth puree.

6. Pour the mango puree into another bowl.

7. Rinse the blender, and now place the raspberries into the blender. Blend the raspberries until you get a smooth puree.

8. Pour the raspberry puree into a third bowl.

9. To assemble the pudding: Take four glasses and pour any one of the fruit purees into the glasses. Make sure that the puree is equally distributed among the glasses.

10. Divide half of the chia pudding among the glasses, and this will be your next layer.

11. Place a tablespoon of yogurt in each glass.

12. Next, pour another fruit puree into the glasses, again distributing equally among the glasses.

13. Divide the third puree equally among the glasses to create the final layer.

14. Sprinkle a tablespoon of hemp seeds on top of each glass.

15. You can serve right away or chill and serve later. If desired, you can garnish with fresh fruit before serving.

Choco-Chip and Banana Pancakes

Number of servings: 6

Nutritional values per serving: (1 pancake)

Calories – 250

Fat – 8 grams

Carbohydrates – 37 grams

Protein – 8 grams

Ingredients:

- 6 tablespoons white self-rising flour
- ½ cup whole-wheat self-rising flour
- 1 tablespoon sugar or coconut sugar or any other sweetener of your choice
- 1 teaspoon baking powder
- 1 overripe banana, mashed
- 1 egg
- ¾ cup + 1/8 cup low-fat or skim milk or almond milk
- 1 teaspoon vanilla extract
- 3 tablespoons chocolate chips
- 1 tablespoon light butter or coconut oil, melted or any other oil of your preference

Serving options:

- Maple syrup or any other syrup of your choice
- Berries
- Coconut butter or nut butter
- Fruit of your choice
- Whipped cream etc.

Directions:

1. Whisk together banana, sugar, vanilla, milk, and egg in a bowl. Add oil and whisk well.

2. Add flour and baking powder and whisk until just incorporated. Add milk and stir until just combined. Do not over-whisk.

3. Add chocolate chips and fold gently.

4. Place a nonstick pan over a medium flame. When the pan is heated, spray the pan with cooking spray. Pour about ¼ cup of batter on the pan. Swirl the pan to spread the pancake. Slowly bubbles will be visible on top. Cook until the underside is brown. Turn the pancake over and cook the other side as well.

5. Remove the pancake from the pan and keep warm.

6. Make the remaining pancakes, similarly, following steps 4 – 5.

7. Serve pancakes with any of the suggested serving options.

Sweet Potato Waffles

Number of servings: 8

Nutritional values per serving: (1 waffle without toppings)

Calories - 270

Fat - 5 grams

Carbohydrates - 52 grams

Protein - 6 grams

Ingredients:

- 1 cup canned sweet potato puree
- 2 tablespoons canola or light olive oil
- 2 tablespoons honey
- 1 cup milk
- 2 eggs
- 2 cups pancake or waffle mix

Directions:

1. Whisk together sweet potatoes, eggs, milk, oil, and honey in a bowl until smooth.

2. Stir in pancake mix using a wooden spoon. Stir until almost free from lumps.

3. Set up your waffle iron and preheat it following the directions of the manufacturer.

4. Pour 1/8 of the batter into the waffle iron. Close the lid and set the timer according to the manufacturer's instructions.

5. Once waffles are cooked, you can serve with toppings of your choice.

6. Cook the remaining waffles similarly. You can store leftover waffles in an airtight container in the refrigerator (good for up to three days). They can be frozen for up to 3 months.

Pink Breakfast Bowl

Number of servings: 2

Nutritional values per serving:

Calories – 365

Fat – 10 grams

Carbohydrates – 54 grams

Protein – 11 grams

Ingredients:

- 1 ½ cups cooked quinoa or millet or rice
- 2 tablespoons raw or lightly toasted seeds like pumpkin seeds or sunflower seeds, or chopped nuts
- 2 cups unsweetened nondairy milk of your choice
- 2 handfuls of dried fruit like raisins, goji berries, and chopped dates
- Hemp seeds to garnish (optional)
- 2 small beets, peeled, finely grated
- 2 tablespoons chia seeds
- 2 teaspoons ground cinnamon

Directions:

1. Combine the cooked quinoa and seeds, milk, beets, chia seeds, and cinnamon in a bowl.
2. Divide into 2 serving bowls.
3. Sprinkle hemp seeds and dried fruit on top and serve.

Chocolate Fudge Brownie Oatmeal

Number of servings: 2

Nutritional values per serving:

Calories – 355

Fat – 6 grams

Carbohydrates – 52 grams

Protein – 27 grams

Ingredients:

- 1 cup old fashioned rolled oats
- Truvia to taste (optional)
- 20 drops stevia extract or to taste
- ¼ cup dark cocoa powder
- 2 cups milk, divided
- 2 scoops of chocolate protein powder

Directions:

1. Place cocoa, oats, truvia, 1 ½ cups milk into a microwave-safe container. Keep stirring until the mixture thickens.

2. Place the container in the microwave and cook on high for about 3 minutes.

3. Combine stevia, ½ cup milk, and protein powder in a bowl. Whisk until free from lumps.

4. Pour into the bowl of oatmeal and keep stirring until well incorporated.

5. Divide into bowls and serve.

Lunch Recipes

Black Beans and Mango Salad

Number of servings: 6

Nutritional values per serving: (about 7 ounces)

Calories – 350

Fat – 1.5 grams

Carbohydrates – 70 grams

Protein – 17 grams

Ingredients:

- 16 ounces cooked or canned black beans
- 2 tablespoons fresh lemon juice
- 2 tablespoons fresh lime juice
- 2 tablespoons orange juice
- 1/3 cup chopped cilantro
- 20 ounces mango, peeled, cut into cubes
- Salt to taste
- 2 tablespoons maple syrup
- Pepper to taste

Directions:

1. Place black beans and mango in a bowl and toss well.
2. Whisk together lime juice, orange juice, and lemon juice in a bowl. Add maple syrup and whisk well. Stir in cilantro, salt, and pepper.
3. Pour over the bean mixture and toss well.
4. Cover the bowl and chill until use.
5. Divide into 6 bowls and serve.

Green Goddess Salad with Chicken

Number of servings: 2

Nutritional values per serving: (about 5 cups with 1 tablespoon of dressing)

Calories – 295

Fat – 7.5 grams

Carbohydrates – 14.5 grams

Protein – 43 grams

Ingredients:

For green goddess dressing:

- 2 avocadoes, peeled, pitted, chopped
- ½ cup fresh, chopped herbs of your choice (you may use a mixture of herbs as well)
- 1 teaspoon salt or to taste
- 3 cups buttermilk
- 4 tablespoons rice vinegar

For salad:

- 6 cups chopped romaine lettuce
- 6 ounces cooked, diced, skinless, boneless chicken breast
- 12 cherry tomatoes, halved
- 2 cups sliced cucumber
- 1 cup diced, low-fat Swiss cheese

Directions:

1. To make green goddess dressing: blend avocado, herbs, salt, buttermilk, and vinegar in a blender until you get a smooth puree. Pour into an airtight container and refrigerate until use. This should make around 3 ½ cups.

2. To serve: drizzle 2 tablespoons dressing over the salad. Stir until well combined.

3. Transfer into two serving bowls. Divide the chicken, tomatoes, and cheese among the bowls. You can add more dressing if desired, and the remaining dressing can be used in some other recipe. It can last for 3 – 4 days in the refrigerator.

4. Serve.

Cucumber Turkey Club Sandwich

Number of servings: 2

Nutritional values per serving: (1 sandwich)

Calories - 325

Fat - 18 grams

Carbohydrates - 15 grams

Protein - 26 grams

Ingredients:

- 2 large cucumbers, peeled, halved lengthwise
- 4 teaspoons mayonnaise
- 2 slices cheddar cheese or Swiss cheese
- 2 thin, round slices of onion
- 4 teaspoons yellow or brown deli mustard
- 4 ounces sliced deli turkey breast
- 6 thin, round slices of tomatoes
- Pepper to taste

Directions:

1. Take a spoon and carefully scoop the seeds from the cucumber halves. Discard the seeds.

2. Spread a teaspoon of mayonnaise and mustard on each half of the cucumber half on the cut side.

3. Place turkey slices on two of the cucumber halves. Layer with cheese, followed by tomatoes and onion. Season with pepper.

4. Complete the sandwich by covering with the remaining cucumber halves.

5. Cut each sandwich into two halves and serve.

Tuna and Chickpea Pita Sandwiches

Number of servings: 2

Nutritional values per serving: (1 sandwich)

Calories – 320

Fat – 8 grams

Carbohydrates – 36 grams

Protein – 23 grams

Ingredients:

For dressing:

- 3 tablespoons fat-free or low-fat Greek yogurt
- 1 ¼ tablespoons fresh lemon juice or to taste
- 1 teaspoon chopped fresh rosemary or ¼ teaspoon dried, crushed rosemary
- 2 tablespoons light mayonnaise
- 1/8 cup chopped fresh parsley
- ½ teaspoon chopped fresh thyme or 1/8 teaspoon dried thyme

For salad sandwich:

- 1 can (4.5 – 5 ounces) white albacore tuna, well-drained
- 6 tablespoons chopped celery
- Salt to taste
- 1 cup chopped spinach
- ½ can (from a 15 ounce can) chickpeas, drained, rinsed
- 3 tablespoons finely chopped red onion
- 1 medium tomato, sliced
- 1 whole wheat pita bread, cut in half

Directions:

1. To make the dressing: combine mayonnaise, Greek yogurt, lemon juice, and herbs in a bowl.

2. To make the salad: combine celery, chickpeas, spinach, onion, and tuna in a bowl. Stir in dressing.

3. To make sandwiches: cut each half of the pita pocket in the center, horizontally (except the edges) to make pockets.

4. Fill the salad and tomatoes into the pita pockets and serve.

Egg Salad Lettuce Wraps

Number of servings: 2

Nutritional values per serving: (2 wraps with 1 cup carrot sticks)

Calories - 435

Fat - 27 grams

Carbohydrates - 21 grams

Protein - 27 grams

Ingredients:

- ½ cup nonfat Greek yogurt
- 1 teaspoon Dijon mustard or to taste
- Salt to taste
- Pepper to taste
- 4 stalks celery, minced
- 4 large iceberg lettuce leaves
- 4 carrots, peeled, cut into sticks
- 2 tablespoons mayonnaise
- Salt to taste
- 6 hard-boiled eggs, peeled,
- ¼ cup minced red onion
- 2 tablespoons chopped fresh basil

Directions:

1. Combine mayonnaise, mustard, yogurt, salt, and pepper in a bowl.

2. Cut the eggs into two halves and remove 2 yolks. These yolks are not needed.

3. Cut all the eggs into cubes. Add eggs into the bowl of mayonnaise along with onion and celery and stir until well combined.

4. Cut each lettuce leaf into two halves. Stack two halves together. You should have four stacks in total.

5. Distribute the egg salad among the lettuce stacks and scatter basil on top. Wrap and serve with carrot sticks.

Cabbage Barley Soup

Number of servings: 4

Nutritional values per serving:

Calories – 195

Fat – 1 grams

Carbohydrates – 37 grams

Protein – 11 grams

Ingredients:

- ¼ cup medium-size pearl barley
- ½ cup dried brown lentils, rinsed
- 1 ½ medium carrots, chopped
- ¼ teaspoon poultry seasoning
- 23 ounces V8 juice
- 4 cups shredded cabbage
- Salt to taste
- 1 stalk celery, chopped
- Pepper to taste
- 2 cups water
- 4 ounces fresh mushrooms, sliced

Directions:

1. Place barley, lentils, carrots, poultry seasoning, V8 juice, water, cabbage, and celery in a soup pot.

2. Place the soup pot over medium flame. When the mixture begins to boil, lower the flame and cook until lentils and barley are tender. It can take a long time to cook, so if you have an instant pot or pressure cooker, use this to make the soup. It will cook much faster.

3. Add salt, pepper, and mushroom and stir. Cover the pot and continue cooking until mushrooms are soft.

4. Ladle into soup bowls and serve.

Carolina Shrimp Soup

Number of servings: 3

Nutritional values per serving:

Calories – 190

Fat – 5 grams

Carbohydrates – 18 grams

Protein – 19 grams

Ingredients:

- 2 teaspoons olive oil, divided
- 3 cloves garlic, minced
- ½ medium sweet red pepper, cut into ¾ inch squares
- ½ can (from a 15.5 ounce can) black-eyed peas, rinsed, drained
- Pepper to taste
- ½ pound uncooked shrimp, peeled, deveined
- ½ bunch kale, trimmed, coarsely chopped (8 cups after chopping)
- 1 ½ cups chicken broth
- Salt to taste
- Finely chopped chives (optional)

Directions:

1. Pour 1 teaspoon oil into a soup pot and heat over medium-high flame. When oil is heated, place shrimp in the pan and stir until they are coated with oil.

2. Stir in garlic and cook for a couple of minutes until they are pink. Transfer the shrimp onto a plate.

3. Pour 1 teaspoon oil into the pot and let it heat. When oil is hot, add kale and red pepper and stir. Cover and cook until the vegetables are tender.

4. Pour broth. When the mixture begins to boil, add black-eyed peas, shrimp, pepper, and salt and stir.

5. Heat thoroughly. Ladle into soup bowls. Garnish with chives and serve.

Sesame Shrimp with Smashed Cucumber Salad

Number of servings: 2

Nutritional values per serving:

Calories – 235

Fat – 15 grams

Carbohydrates – 9 grams

Protein – 16 grams

Ingredients:

- 2 tablespoons toasted sesame oil, divided
- 2 ½ teaspoons low-sodium soy sauce, divided
- 1 tablespoon chopped flat-leaf parsley
- ½ tablespoon honey
- ½ teaspoon crushed red pepper
- ½ pound medium shrimp, peeled, deveined
- 1 cup thinly sliced cucumber
- 1 tablespoon rice vinegar
- ½ tablespoon minced fresh ginger
- 2 small cloves garlic, minced

Directions:

1. Pour a tablespoon of oil into a skillet and heat over medium-high flame. Add shrimp once the oil is hot. Cook for 3 minutes, flip, and cook the other side for 3 minutes.

2. Stir in 1 ½ teaspoons soy sauce and cook for about 30 seconds. Turn off the heat.

3. Pour remaining oil and soy sauce into a Ziploc bag. Also, add parsley, honey, red pepper, cucumber, rice vinegar, ginger, and garlic.

4. Seal the bag. Shake well so that the contents are well combined.

5. Place the bag on your cutting board so that it is lying flat. Roll the bag with a rolling pin. This is done to smash the cucumber slices.

6. Divide shrimp onto two plates. Divide the cucumber mixture onto the plates and serve.

Quinoa Corn Chowder

Number of servings: 4

Nutritional values per serving:

Calories – 315

Fat – 9 grams

Carbohydrates – 48 grams

Protein – 12 grams

Ingredients:

- ½ cup quinoa
- ½ medium onion, diced
- ½ teaspoon minced garlic
- ¼ teaspoon dried thyme
- ½ teaspoon dried parsley
- 2 tablespoons flour
- 1 cup milk
- ½ can (from a 15 ounce can) white kidney beans, rinsed, drained
- 1 ½ tablespoons canola oil
- ½ red pepper, diced
- Salt to taste
- 1 ½ cups chicken broth
- 2 cups fresh or frozen corn kernels

Directions:

1. Place a pot over a medium flame. Let the pot heat up. Add quinoa and toast for 2 to 3 minutes until you get a nice aroma. Keep stirring throughout.

2. Stir in oil, pepper, and onion and raise the heat to medium-high.

3. Cook until the onion turns translucent. Stir in garlic, salt, and dried herbs. Cook for about a minute or until you get a nice fragrance.

4. Add flour and stir until well incorporated. Add broth and whisk well.

5. Add milk, stirring constantly. Keep stirring until slightly thick and comes to a boil.

6. Lower the flame and cook without covering until quinoa is tender.

7. Stir in the corn and beans. Heat thoroughly.

8. Ladle into soup bowls and serve.

Oven-Fried Chicken

Number of servings: 2

Nutritional values per serving:

Calories – 320

Fat – 14 grams

Carbohydrates – 24 grams

Protein – 21 grams

Ingredients:

- ½ pound frozen chicken breasts, thawed, cut into strips
- 6 tablespoons flour
- ¼ teaspoon salt
- 1 teaspoon paprika
- ¼ teaspoon pepper
- 2 tablespoons melted butter or more if required
- ¼ cup panko breadcrumbs
- ½ tablespoon seasoning salt

Directions:

1. Line a baking tray by placing a sheet of parchment paper over it. Brush butter on the parchment paper as well.

2. Place flour, salt, pepper, paprika, breadcrumbs, and salt in a Ziploc bag. Seal the bag and shake until well combined.

3. Place chicken in the bag and seal the bag. Shake until the chicken is coated with the mixture.

4. Place the coated chicken on the baking sheet. Make sure to space out the strips.

5. Place the baking tray in an oven that has been preheated to 425°F and bake for about 10 minutes.

6. Flip the chicken over and continue baking for 10 – 15 minutes or until the chicken is cooked through and golden-brown on the outside.

7. Serve right away.

Greek Salad Wraps

Number of servings: 3

Nutritional values per serving: (1 wrap with 1 ½ cups of salad)

Calories – 335

Fat – 14 grams

Carbohydrates – 42 grams

Protein – 9 grams

Ingredients:

- 3 tablespoons red wine vinegar
- 1 tablespoon finely chopped fresh oregano
- Salt to taste
- Pepper to taste
- ½ can (from a 15 ounce can) low-sodium chickpeas, rinsed
- ½ cup halved cherry tomatoes or grape tomatoes
- 1/8 cup slivered red onion
- 2 tablespoons extra-virgin olive oil
- 4 cups chopped romaine lettuce
- ¾ cup sliced cucumbers (cut into half-moon slices)
- 1/8 cup sliced, pitted kalamata olives
- 3 whole-wheat wraps (8 – 9 inches each)

Directions:

1. Combine oil, vinegar, pepper, salt, and oregano in a large bowl. Whisk well.

2. Add all the vegetables, chickpeas, and olives and toss well.

3. Spread the wraps on a large serving plate. Divide the salad among the wraps (each portion should be 1 ½ cups).

4. Roll the wraps and place with the seam side facing down.

Snack Recipes

Mini Chicken Fajitas

Number of servings: 18

Nutritional values per serving: (1 mini fajita)

Calories - 40

Fat - 2 grams

Carbohydrates - 3 grams

Protein - 3 grams

Ingredients:

- 1 tablespoon oil of your choice
- ½ yellow bell pepper, cut into ½ inch squares
- ½ red bell pepper, cut into ½ inch squares
- 1 skinless chicken breast, cut into ½ inch squares
- ½ teaspoon ground coriander
- ½ teaspoon ground cumin
- 1/8 teaspoon chili powder or to taste
- 8 ounces canned, chopped tomatoes
- 2 green onions, thinly sliced
- 3 small flour tortillas
- 1 tablespoon chipotle paste
- A handful of fresh cilantro, chopped
- 1.5 ounces pre-grated mozzarella cheese

For guacamole:

- ½ avocado, peeled, pitted, mashed
- 2 small cloves garlic, crushed
- Juice of ½ lime or more to taste
- 1 tablespoon finely chopped fresh cilantro

Directions:

1. Pour oil into a nonstick pan and heat over medium flame. When the oil is heated, add chicken and bell peppers and cook for a couple of minutes.

2. Combine cumin, coriander, and chili powder in a bowl and sprinkle over the chicken and peppers. Stir-fry for a few more seconds.

3. Add tomatoes and chipotle paste and mix well. Cook until you get a nice and thick sauce. Make sure you stir often.

4. Add green onions and cilantro and mix well. Turn off the flame after a minute. Let cool.

5. Meanwhile, cut each tortilla into six equal triangles, so you get 18 triangles in total.

6. Take a teaspoonful of the chicken mixture and place it on the shorter end of the triangle. Place a little of the cheese over the chicken mixture.

7. Now start rolling from this side, along with the filling, till you reach the tip of the triangle. Insert a toothpick to fasten and place it on a baking tray.

8. Repeat steps 6 – 7 and make the remaining fajitas.

9. Cover the baking tray with plastic wrap and place it in the refrigerator until use.

10. Meanwhile, to make guacamole, combine avocado, garlic, lime juice, and cilantro in a bowl and stir until smooth. Cover and place in the refrigerator until use. Use the dip within two days.

11. To cook the fajitas, remove the plastic wrap and place the baking tray in an oven that has been preheated to 350°F, for about 10 minutes or until nice and hot.

12. Serve mini fajitas with guacamole.

Hummus

Number of servings: 3

Nutritional values per serving: (4 tablespoons)

Calories – 145

Fat – 9 grams

Carbohydrates – 13 grams

Protein – 3 grams

Ingredients:

- 2 small cloves garlic, peeled, smashed, finely chopped
- 1 ½ tablespoons fresh lemon juice
- ½ tablespoon tahini
- ½ can (from a 15 ounce can) chickpeas, rinsed, drained
- 1 ½ tablespoons extra-virgin olive oil
- ¼ teaspoon salt

Directions:

1. Place garlic, chickpeas, olive oil, lemon juice, salt, and tahini in the food processor bowl. Keep blending until you get a smooth puree.

2. Pour into a bowl. Cover the bowl and chill until use. It can last for five days.

3. You can serve hummus with vegetable sticks (carrots, cucumber, celery, etc.), crackers, or falafel. You can also use it with pita chips or as a filling or spread for sandwiches. You can also use it in salads.

Easy Oven Baked Falafel

Number of servings: 2

Nutritional values per serving: (3 falafels, without hummus or other serving options)

Calories – 155

Fat – 1 gram

Carbohydrates – 25 grams

Protein – 6 grams

Ingredients:

- ¾ cup cooked or canned chickpeas
- ½ cup parsley
- 2 cloves garlic, peeled
- 1 tablespoon lime juice
- ½ teaspoon sea salt
- ½ teaspoon basil
- ¼ teaspoon ground nutmeg
- ½ cup chopped cilantro
- 2 tablespoons whole-wheat flour
- ¼ red onion, finely chopped
- ½ teaspoon pepper
- ½ teaspoon ground cumin
- ½ teaspoon dried oregano

Directions:

1. Place herbs, spices, lime juice, chickpeas, garlic, and onion in the food processor bowl and process until you get a coarse mixture.

2. Add whole wheat flour and give short pulses until well combined, and you get a sticky dough.

3. Add the mixture into a bowl. Place the bowl in the refrigerator for about 30 minutes.

4. Prepare a baking tray by lining it with parchment paper. Make six equal portions of the mixture and shape them into patties.

5. Place the patties on the baking tray and put it in an oven that has been preheated to 425°F for about 30 – 40 minutes or baked until crisp and brown.

6. Serve falafel with hummus. You can also make a bigger falafel and place it in between buns with toppings of your choice to make falafel burgers. You can stuff it in pita bread along with hummus and vegetables to make sandwiches.

Apple Pie Energy Bites

Number of servings: 12

Nutritional values per serving: (2 bites)

Calories – 320

Fat – 15 grams

Carbohydrates – 39 grams

Protein – 9 g

Ingredients:

- 4 cups old fashioned rolled oats
- 4 tablespoons ground flaxseeds
- 2 tablespoons chopped hazelnuts
- 1 teaspoon ground allspice
- 2 teaspoons vanilla extract
- ½ cup unsweetened dried cranberries
- 2 teaspoons ground cinnamon
- 1 teaspoon salt
- 2 tablespoons chopped walnuts
- 1 cup almond butter
- 4 tablespoons honey
- 2 cups grated Granny Smith apples
- 2 teaspoons lemon juice

Directions:

1. Place apples in a bowl. Drizzle lemon juice all over and toss well.

2. Combine oats, flaxseeds, cinnamon, salt, nuts, and allspice in another bowl.

3. Combine honey, vanilla, and almond butter in a third bowl.

4. Pour the honey mixture into the bowl of oats and stir until well incorporated.

5. Add apples and cranberries and stir until well incorporated.

6. Divide the mixture into 24 equal portions and shape into balls. Place the balls in an airtight container and chill until use. It can last for 4 days.

Chipotle Black Bean Dip with Corn Chips

Number of servings: 3

Nutritional values per serving: (6 tortilla chips with ¼ cup dip)

Calories – 145

Fat – 3.5 grams

Carbohydrates – 28 grams

Protein – 6.5 grams

Ingredients:

- 3 corn tortillas (6 inches each), cut each into 6 equal wedges
- ½ teaspoon olive oil
- ½ teaspoon cumin seeds
- Salt to taste
- ½ cup chopped onions
- 2 small cloves garlic, minced
- ½ can (from a 15 ounce can) black beans, with its liquid
- 1 tablespoon crumbled queso fresco cheese
- ½ chipotle chili in adobo sauce
- A large pinch dried oregano
- ½ ounce shredded part-skim mozzarella cheese
- 3 tablespoons unsalted, canned, diced tomatoes with its liquid

Directions:

1. Take a baking tray and cover with a sheet of parchment paper, and grease it with cooking spray. Place wedges on the baking sheet. Season with salt.

2. Place the baking tray in an oven that has been preheated to 400°F and bake for about 10 minutes or until crisp and brown. Make sure to flip the tortilla chips halfway through baking.

3. While the chips are baking, pour oil into a saucepan and place the saucepan over medium flame.

4. When the oil is heated, add onion and cook until translucent. Stir in cumin and garlic and sauté for a minute or until you get a nice aroma.

5. Stir in beans and oregano and mash well using a potato masher.

6. Lower the flame and cook until thick. Turn off the flame.

7. Grease a small baking dish with cooking spray. Spread the bean mixture into the baking dish.

8. Sprinkle queso fresco and mozzarella cheese on top. Place the baking dish in the oven and bake for a few minutes until cheese melts and is bubbling.

9. Blend together tomatoes and chipotle chili into a blender until you get a smooth puree.

10. Pour the tomato mixture over the cheese layer. Garnish with cilantro and serve with corn chips.

Almond Poppy Crackers

Number of servings: 40

Nutritional values per serving: (1 cracker)

Calories – 60

Fat – 5 grams

Carbohydrates – 2 grams

Protein – 2 grams

Ingredients:

- 3 cups almond flour
- 2 tablespoons olive oil
- 2 large egg whites
- 2 tablespoons poppy seeds
- 2 teaspoons fine grain salt

Directions:

1. Prepare two baking trays by lining them with parchment paper. Keep rack in the center of the oven. Set the temperature of the oven to 350°F and preheat the oven.

2. Place almond flour, salt, and poppy seeds in a bowl and stir until well combined.

3. Stir in oil and egg whites. Mix until a dough is formed. Divide the dough into 2 equal portions and shape it into balls.

4. Place a dough ball on the center of the baking tray. Place another sheet of parchment paper on top of the dough. Roll with a rolling pin, giving the shape of an 8 x 12 inches rectangle.

5. Gently remove the top parchment paper. Cut into 20 equal rectangles. Do not separate the crackers yet.

6. Repeat steps 4 – 5 and make the remaining crackers.

7. Bake the crackers in batches.

8. Place the baking sheet in an oven that has been preheated to 350°F for about 12 – 14 minutes or until crisp and brown. Keep watch over the crackers after 12 minutes of baking as they can burn easily.

9. Let cool completely. You can now separate the crackers by either breaking them apart or cutting them once again on the marked rectangles.

10. Transfer the crackers into an airtight container. It can last for a week. You can serve the crackers as is or with a dip or toppings of your choice.

Frozen Berry Yogurt

Number of servings: 2

Nutritional values per serving:

Calories – 70

Fat – 0 grams

Carbohydrates – 10 grams

Protein – 7 grams

Ingredients:

- 4.4 ounces frozen mixed berries
- ½ tablespoon honey or agave nectar
- 4.4 ounces nonfat Greek yogurt

Directions:

1. Place berries in the food processor bowl along with honey and yogurt. Blend until you get a soft-serve texture.

2. Serve in bowls right away.

Turkey Pesto Roll-Up

Number of servings: 4

Nutritional values per serving: (3 rolls)

Calories – 165

Fat – 7.5 grams

Carbohydrates – 11.5 grams

Protein – 12 grams

Ingredients:

- 2 cucumbers (about 6 – 7 inches long), trimmed, unpeeled
- 2 ounces cheddar cheese (6 thin slices)
- 2 red bell peppers, cut into matchsticks
- 4 ounces deli turkey (6 thin slices)
- 2 tablespoons pesto or more if required
- Pepper to taste
- 2 cups greens of your choice
- Salt and pepper to taste

Directions:

1. Cut the cucumbers into thin slices with a mandoline slicer or a sharp knife. You should get about six slices from each cucumber.

2. Spread pesto lightly on the cucumber slices. Place turkey slices and cheese slices over the cucumber slices. Sprinkle with salt and pepper. Spread the thin bell pepper slices and greens over the cheese.

3. Roll the cucumber slices and fasten with a toothpick.

4. Serve.

Tomato Basil Soup

Number of servings: 6

Nutritional values per serving:

Calories - 80

Fat - 4 grams

Carbohydrates - 9 grams

Protein - 3 grams

Ingredients:

- 4 teaspoons olive oil
- 2 stalks celery, finely chopped
- 1 cup chopped fresh basil
- 4 cans (14 ounces each) diced tomatoes, unsalted
- 2 small onions, finely chopped
- 2 cloves garlic, peeled, minced
- 2 teaspoons chopped fresh thyme
- Salt to taste
- 4 cups vegetable broth or chicken broth
- Pepper to taste

Directions:

1. Pour oil into a soup pot and place it over medium flame. When the oil is heated, add onion, garlic, and celery and cook until slightly tender. Make sure that the garlic does not turn brown.

2. Stir in the herbs, broth, and tomatoes. When it starts to boil, lower the flame and cook for about 15 minutes, stirring every 5 minutes. Turn off the flame and let it cool.

3. Blend the soup using an immersion blender until smooth or to the desired consistency. You can use a regular blender.

4. Serve the soup hot, warm, or chilled.

Zucchini Feta Fritters

Number of servings: 4

Nutritional values per serving: (3 fritters)

Calories - 240

Fat - 9 grams

Carbohydrates - 24 grams

Protein - 17 grams

Ingredients:

- 2 pounds zucchini, trimmed, peeled, shredded
- ½ cup finely chopped parsley
- ½ cup finely chopped dill
- 2 eggs
- Salt to taste
- 1 cup feta cheese crumbles
- 2 jalapeño peppers, diced
- ½ cup flour or more if required
- Pepper to taste

Directions:

1. Place zucchini on a large cheesecloth. Bring the edges together and squeeze out the moisture, removing as much as possible.

2. Place zucchini, parsley, dill, eggs, salt, feta cheese, jalapeño peppers, flour, and pepper in a bowl and mix until well combined. If the mixture is watery, add more flour and mix well.

3. Divide the mixture into 12 equal portions and form it into patties.

4. Place a large nonstick pan over a medium flame. Spray the pan with cooking spray. Place fritters in the pan (as many as can fit) and fry the remaining in batches.

5. Cook until the underside is golden brown. Flip the fritters over and cook the other side until golden brown.

6. Remove the fritters from the pan and place them on a plate.

7. Cook the remaining fritters similarly.

8. Serve fritters with tzatziki or yogurt sauce. The recipe of tzatziki follows in the next recipe (Mediterranean meatballs gyro sandwich).

Dinner Recipes

Mediterranean Meatballs Gyro Sandwich

Number of servings: 2

Nutritional values per serving:

Calories – 345

Fat – 14.5 grams

Carbohydrates – 21 grams

Protein – 31 grams

Ingredients:

For tzatziki sauce:

- ½ cup Greek yogurt
- ½ teaspoon finely minced garlic
- ½ tablespoon finely chopped fresh dill
- 1/8 teaspoon freshly cracked black pepper
- 1/8 cup grated English cucumber
- ½ teaspoon extra-virgin olive oil
- Sea salt to taste
- ½ tablespoon fresh lemon juice

For Mediterranean meatballs:

- 1/8 cup crushed pork rinds
- 1 tablespoon chopped, fresh flat-leaf parsley
- ¼ teaspoon ground cumin
- Freshly cracked pepper
- 1 small egg
- ½ tablespoon finely minced garlic
- ¼ teaspoon sea salt or to taste
- ½ pound ground chuck

For salad:

- ½ cup finely diced tomatoes
- ½ tablespoon finely chopped flat-leaf parsley
- ½ cup finely diced English cucumber
- Salt to taste
- ¼ cup finely chopped red onion
- Pepper to taste

To assemble:

- 2 flatbreads
- A handful of chopped parsley to garnish
- Crumbled feta cheese (optional)

Directions:

1. To make tzatziki sauce: Place yogurt, garlic, cucumber, dill, oil, pepper, lemon juice, and salt in a bowl and stir until well combined.

2. Cover the bowl and chill in the fridge until use.

3. Place a rack on a baking tray. Spray cooking spray on the rack.

4. Set the oven temperature to 425°F to preheat.

5. To make Mediterranean meatballs: mix together the pork rinds, raw egg, parsley, cumin, garlic, salt, and pepper in a bowl.

6. Add the meat and mix by hand until well combined. Make sure you do not over-mix, or else the meat will become tough.

7. Make eight equal meatballs of the mixture and place them on the rack.

8. Place the rack along with the baking tray in the oven and bake for 10 – 15 minutes or until well-cooked inside. There should be no pink in the middle. Let the meatballs rest on your countertop for 5 minutes.

9. To make the salad: combine tomatoes, cucumber, parsley, and onions in a bowl. Season with salt and pepper.

10. To assemble the sandwich: set up the oven to broil mode. Take a baking sheet and keep the flatbreads on it.

11. Place baking sheet in the oven and broil for a few minutes until toasted lightly. Turn the flatbreads over and broil for a couple of minutes until toasted lightly.

12. To assemble: place four meatballs along the diameter of each flatbread. Spread tzatziki sauce around the meatballs. Be generous with the tzatziki.

13. Scatter the salad over the meatballs. Sprinkle parsley and feta cheese. Roll the flatbreads and place on a serving plate with the seam side down, then serve.

Turkey Chili

Number of servings: 3

Nutritional values per serving: (1-½ cups, without serving options)

Calories – 335

Fat – 4 grams

Carbohydrates – 46 grams

Protein – 32 grams

Ingredients:

- 1 teaspoon olive oil
- 2 cloves garlic, minced
- ½ pound extra-lean (99%) ground turkey or chicken
- 1 teaspoon ground cumin
- 1/8 teaspoon cayenne pepper
- 2 tablespoons chili powder
- ½ teaspoon dried oregano
- Salt to taste
- ¾ cup chicken broth
- ½ can (from a 15 ounce can) sweet corn, rinsed, drained
- ½ can (from a 28 ounce can) diced tomatoes or crushed tomatoes
- ½ red bell pepper, diced
- 1 can (15 ounce can) dark red kidney beans, rinsed, and drained

Optional toppings:

- Grated cheese
- Tortilla chips
- Sour cream
- Chopped cilantro
- Chopped avocado

- Any other toppings of your choice

Directions:

1. Pour oil into a soup pot and place it over medium-high flame. When the oil is heated, add garlic, onion, and red bell pepper and cook for a few minutes until slightly tender.

2. Stir in turkey. Cook until the meat is light brown. As you stir, break down the turkey into smaller pieces.

3. Stir in the spices, salt, and oregano, and cook for a few seconds until you get a nice aroma.

4. Stir in tomatoes, kidney beans, broth, and corn. When it begins to boil, lower the flame and cook until thick. Stir occasionally.

5. Taste the chili and adjust seasoning as required.

6. Ladle into bowls. Serve with any of the suggested serving options.

Chicken Chow Mein

Number of servings: 3

Nutritional values per serving:

Calories – 390

Fat – 5 grams

Carbohydrates – 59 grams

Protein – 24 grams

Ingredients:

- ½ tablespoon canola oil
- ½ red bell pepper, diced
- 1 ½ cups shredded cabbage or coleslaw mix
- ½ teaspoon minced garlic
- A pinch of red pepper flakes
- 2 tablespoons soy sauce
- 6.6 ounces whole-wheat spaghetti
- ½ tablespoon cornstarch mixed with a tablespoon of water (optional)
- 1 ½ chicken breasts, skinless, boneless, cut into cubes
- ½ cup stringed snap peas
- 1 large carrot, peeled, shredded
- ¼ teaspoon minced ginger
- 2 cups chicken broth
- 2 tablespoons hoisin sauce

Directions:

1. Place a pot over a medium-high flame. Add oil and let it heat. Once the oil is heated, add chicken and cook until brown.

2. Stir in peas, red pepper, carrot, and cabbage, and cook until slightly tender.

3. Stir in ginger, garlic, and red pepper flakes. Cook for a few seconds until you get a nice aroma.

4. Pour soy sauce, broth, and hoisin sauce and mix well. When the mixture begins to boil, lower the heat to medium and add in the pasta.

5. Stir often and cook until nearly dry. Now cover the pot and continue cooking for a couple of minutes or until pasta is cooked.

6. Add cornstarch mixture if desired and constantly stir until thick.

7. Serve hot.

Chicken Tortilla Soup

Number of servings: 4

Nutritional values per serving:

Calories – 200

Fat – 8 grams

Carbohydrates – 9 grams

Protein – 22 grams

Ingredients:

- 1 tablespoon olive oil
- ½ can (from a 4 ounce can) chopped green chilies
- ½ jalapeño, chopped
- ½ can (from a 15 ounce can) tomato sauce
- 2 ½ cups low sodium chicken broth
- 2 tablespoons minced cilantro
- Salt to taste
- Pepper to taste
- ½ large onion, chopped
- 1 clove garlic, minced
- ½ teaspoon ground cumin
- ½ can (from a 14.5 ounce can) diced tomatoes with garlic and onion, with its liquid
- ½ rotisserie chicken, shredded, skinless
- 1 teaspoon lime juice
- Shredded Monterey Jack or sharp cheddar cheese to serve
- Crushed tortilla chips to serve

Directions:

1. Place a Dutch oven over medium flame. Add oil and let it heat. Add onions once the oil is hot and cook until they turn soft.

2. Stir in garlic, chili, cumin, and jalapeño. Stir constantly for about a minute or until you get a nice aroma.

3. Add tomatoes, tomato sauce, and broth. Stir well and wait for it to come to a boil.

4. Lower the flame and add chicken. Mix well. Cook for about 7 – 8 minutes.

5. Stir in lime juice, cilantro, salt, and pepper.

6. Ladle into soup bowls. Garnish with tortilla chips, cheese, and serve.

Maple Glazed Salmon

Number of servings: 2

Nutritional values per serving: (1 fillet)

Calories – 270

Fat – 9.5 grams

Carbohydrates – 7 grams

Protein – 36 grams

Ingredients:

- 2 skinless salmon fillets (6 ounces each)
- ¼ – ½ teaspoon garlic powder
- ¼ teaspoon smoked paprika
- ¼ teaspoon salt
- A pinch of ground red pepper
- Lemon juice to drizzle

Directions:

1. Set the oven to broil mode and preheat the oven to high heat. Prepare a baking tray by lining it with aluminum foil. Spray cooking spray over the foil.

2. Mix salt and all the spices in a bowl. Sprinkle spice mixture all over the fillets and place them on the baking tray.

3. Place baking tray in the oven. Set the timer for 5 minutes and let the fillets broil.

4. Brush maple syrup over the fillets and broil for another minute or until the fish is the way you like it cooked (ideal temperature for salmon is medium-rare to medium).

5. Squeeze lemon juice on top and serve.

Vegetarian Bourguignon

Number of servings: 2 - 3

Nutritional values per serving: (1 cup)

Calories - 270

Fat - 10 grams

Carbohydrates - 23 grams

Protein - 4 grams

Ingredients:

- 1 ½ tablespoons butter, divided
- 1 stalk celery, sliced
- ½ cup chopped carrots (½ inch pieces)
- ½ large shallot, minced
- 2 small bay leaves
- ½ cup chopped parsnip (½ inch pieces)
- ½ pound mixed mushrooms, halved
- 2 small cloves garlic, minced
- ½ tablespoon extra-virgin olive oil
- ¼ teaspoon dried thyme
- Salt to taste
- Pepper to taste
- ½ tablespoon all-purpose flour
- 2 tablespoons cognac or brandy
- ¾ cup frozen pearl onions, thawed
- 1 tablespoon tomato paste
- ¾ cup dry red wine
- ¾ cup vegetable broth or mushroom broth

Directions:

1.Place a pot over a medium-high flame. Add 1 tablespoon of butter and ½ a tablespoon of oil. When the butter melts, stir in the parsnip, celery, and carrot and cook until the veggies are slightly tender.

2.Lower the heat to medium and stir in the shallot, mushrooms, bay leaves, salt, garlic, thyme, and pepper, and cook until the mushrooms are soft.

3.Add tomato paste and mix well. Scatter flour on top and constantly stir for about 30 seconds.

4.Pour wine and cognac and stir. Raise to medium-high heat and scrape the bottom of the pot to remove any particles that may be stuck. When the liquid in the pot reduces to half its original quantity, stir in the broth.

5.When the mixture begins to boil, lower the flame once again and cover the pot partially. Let it simmer until the vegetables are slightly soft.

6.Add pearl onions and stir. Continue cooking for another 4 – 5 minutes.

7.Turn off the heat. Add ½ a tablespoon of butter, salt, and pepper and stir.

8.Serve hot.

Vegetarian Enchilada Casserole

Number of servings: 4

Nutritional values per serving: (1 ½ cups)

Calories – 360

Fat – 17 grams

Carbohydrates – 42 grams

Protein – 14 grams

Ingredients:

- 1 tablespoon extra-virgin olive oil
- 6 tablespoons chopped poblano peppers
- ½ medium zucchini halved lengthwise, cut into ¼ inch thick half moons
- ½ medium yellow squash halved lengthwise, cut into ¼ inch half moons
- ½ cup chopped onion
- 3 cloves garlic, minced
- ½ cup fresh corn kernels
- ¼ teaspoon salt or to taste
- ½ can (from a 15 ounce can) unsalted black beans, rinsed
- ½ can (from a 15 ounce can) unsalted pinto beans, rinsed
- 4 corn tortillas (6 inches each)
- ½ avocado, peeled, pitted, diced
- ¼ cup low-fat sour cream
- ½ cup Pico de Gallo
- ¼ teaspoon salt or to taste
- ¾ cup shredded pepper Jack cheese
- ¼ cup sliced scallions

Directions:

1. Pour oil into a skillet and heat over medium-high flame. When the oil is heated, add onion, garlic, and poblano peppers and cook for a few minutes.

2. When the onion turns pink, stir in zucchini, squash, Pico de Gallo, corn, and salt. Cook until slightly thick.

3. Turn off the heat. Add pinto and black beans. Stir until well combined.

4. Grease a small baking dish or casserole dish with cooking spray.

5. Spread 1/3 of the bean mixture into the baking dish.

6. Spread two tortillas over the bean mixture. If needed, tear the tortillas to fit into the dish.

7. Repeat steps 5 - 6. Spread the remaining bean mixture over the tortillas. Finally, top with cheese.

8. Set the oven temperature to 350°F to preheat. Place the baking dish in the oven and bake for about 20 - 25 minutes until heated thoroughly and the cheese melts.

9. Garnish with sour cream, scallions, and avocado.

10. Serve.

Ham and Pineapple Rice

Number of servings: 2

Nutritional values per serving:

Calories – 330

Fat – 3 grams

Carbohydrates – 60 grams

Protein – 17 grams

Ingredients:

- 1 cup cooked, chopped ham
- ½ can (from a 13.2 ounce can) pineapple tidbits, drained but retaining the juice
- 1 tablespoon soy sauce
- ¼ teaspoon salt or to taste
- 1 green onion, sliced
- ¾ cup low-sodium chicken broth
- ½ tablespoon Worcestershire sauce
- ½ cup long-grain white or brown rice rinsed well
- ¼ cup pineapple juice or more if required (use the juice from the canned pineapple)

Directions:

1. Place ham, pineapple juice, Worcestershire sauce, soy sauce, broth, and salt in a skillet. Place the skillet over high flame.

2. When the mixture begins to boil, add raw rice and stir. Lower the heat to medium-low. Cook covered until dry. If the rice looks uncooked, add more of the pineapple juice and simmer until rice is cooked.

3. Add green onions, stir, and serve.

Skillet Chicken Parmesan

Number of servings: 2

Nutritional values per serving:

Calories – 440

Fat – 24 grams

Carbohydrates – 11 grams

Protein – 46 grams

Ingredients:

- 2 boneless, skinless chicken breasts
- Salt to taste
- ½ teaspoon minced garlic
- ½ teaspoon dried oregano
- ½ teaspoon dried parsley
- Pepper to taste
- ½ can (from a 28 ounce can) crushed tomatoes
- ½ teaspoon sugar (optional)
- ¼ cup shredded parmesan cheese
- ¼ cup shredded mozzarella cheese
- 1 tablespoon canola oil
- 1 small onion, chopped

Directions:

1. Pour oil into a skillet and place the skillet over a medium flame. Let the oil heat.

2. Season chicken with salt and pepper and place in the skillet.

3. Cook until golden brown all over and well-cooked inside.

4. Remove chicken from the pan and place it on a plate to rest. Keep the plate covered with aluminum foil.

5. Add onion into the skillet and cook until soft. Stir in the garlic and herbs. Cook for about a minute or until you get a nice aroma.

6. Throw in the salt, tomatoes, and sugar. Cook over medium-low flame for about 5 minutes.

7. Place the chicken back in the pan and stir. Heat thoroughly. Turn off the heat. Sprinkle cheese on top and cover the pan with a lid for a few minutes until the cheese melts.

8. Serve.

Skillet Lasagna

Number of servings: 10

Nutritional values per serving:

Calories – 430

Fat – 9 grams

Carbohydrates – 51 grams

Protein – 38 grams

Ingredients:

- 2 pounds ground turkey or chicken or lean ground beef
- 1 onion, finely chopped
- 2 small zucchinis, trimmed, shredded
- 2 bell peppers, chopped
- 2 large carrots, shredded
- Pepper to taste
- Salt to taste
- 2 teaspoons Italian seasoning
- Red pepper flakes to taste
- 6 cups low-sodium chicken broth
- 2 cups shredded mozzarella cheese
- 2 cans (14 ounces each) crushed tomatoes
- 17.5 ounces dry lasagna sheets

Directions:

1. Place a skillet over a medium flame. Add turkey and cook until light brown. Break the meat as it cooks.

2. Stir in the onion and pepper. Once the turkey turns brown, stir in the zucchini, carrots, and spices.

3. Add in the broth and tomatoes and mix well. Add the lasagna sheets into the skillet and place them in layers with turkey and vegetables between each one, making sure the lasagna is coated by the broth and tomatoes.

4. Increase the heat to medium-high and cook until the pasta is al dente. Turn off the heat.

5. Garnish with cheese and cover the pot. Let it rest for 5 minutes. Serve right away.

Sample Meal Plan

Now that you are armed with all the recipes you need to follow the 16/8 intermittent fasting protocol, it is time to create a meal plan. Here is a sample meal plan that you can use for inspiration:

Day 1

Breakfast: Peanut butter cup shake.

Lunch: Green goddess salad with chicken.

Dinner: Skillet Chicken Parmesan.

Day 2

Breakfast: Veggie mini quiches.

Lunch: Black bean and mango salad.

Dinner: Maple-glazed salmon.

Day 3

Breakfast: Dark chocolate peppermint shake.

Lunch: Tuna and chickpea pita sandwiches.

Dinner: Vegetarian bourguignon.

Day 4

Breakfast: Ham, egg, and avocado breakfast burrito.

Lunch: Cucumber turkey club sandwiches.

Dinner: Chicken tortilla soup.

Day 5

Breakfast: Very berry super shake.

Lunch: Egg salad lettuce wraps.

Dinner: Chicken chow mein.

Day 6

Breakfast: Cauliflower English muffins.

Lunch: Cabbage barley soup.

Dinner: Turkey chili.

Day 7

Breakfast: Summer skillet vegetables and egg scramble.

Lunch: Carolina shrimp soup.

Dinner: Mediterranean meatballs gyro sandwich.

Conclusion

Ultimately, intermittent fasting is incredibly simple. The 16/8 protocol suggests you need to fast for sixteen hours a day, with an eating window restricted to only eight hours. Depending on your needs and requirements, you can easily accommodate several meals and snacks within this timeframe. All your nutritional requirements can be fulfilled without compromising taste. Also, since intermittent fasting doesn't explicitly exclude any food groups, you can add various meals to your daily diet.

Don't forget to include some form of physical activity in your daily schedule if you want to enhance and maintain the benefits of intermittent fasting. Whether weight loss is your priority or you want to improve your overall health, this diet has something to offer for everyone. Since it is perfectly sustainable, you can reap all the benefits it has to offer in weeks. By following the simple advice and suggestions given in this book, transitioning into this form of eating becomes easy. While making a dietary change, make sure you are mentally and physically ready for it. Don't hesitate to use the intermittent fasting tips, strategies, and suggestions in this book to maximize your chances of success.

Before you jump headfirst into this diet, make sure you know why you are doing it. This motivation will help you to overcome any setbacks you face while fasting.

So, what are you waiting for? All that's left is to create an action plan and get going. By simply paying attention to when you eat, you can improve your overall health and wellbeing. The key to good health lies in your hands. Don't forget to stock your pantry with all the required ingredients to cook delicious, healthy, and filling intermittent fasting recipes. Coupled with a helpful meal plan, this will make following the diet quite simple. Once you get into the groove of intermittent fasting, and with a good dose of perseverance and determination, you will notice substantial improvements in your overall health and wellbeing!

Part 2: Intermittent Fasting for Women Over 50

The One-Stop Guide to Lose Weight, Slow Down Aging, and Support Your Hormones While Still Enjoying Delicious Meals and Social Gatherings

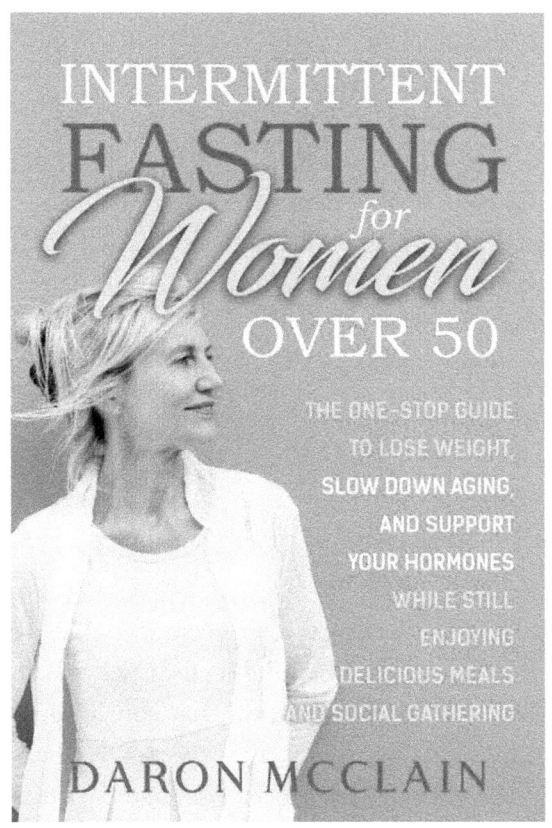

Introduction

Intermittent fasting (IF) was named the "trendiest" weight loss term searched on Google in 2019 and was featured in the New England Journal of Medicine. These two things happened for a reason. This diet method had quickly become one of the most popular among dieters. Anyone who is a part of the weight loss and fitness world likely knows what it entails.

Intermittent fasting involves alternate fasting and eating cycles. You have periods when you eat and periods when you fast. There have been many proven benefits, such as weight loss, health improvement, and disease protection. Another possible advantage is that it could help you live longer.

Naturally, there are tons of resources available online to teach people how to practice intermittent fasting. Still, not all these resources include factual information that can improve your health and life quality. This is precisely why Intermittent Fasting for Women over 50 exists. This book has been written explicitly to target women in their 50s or their menopausal stage of life.

It is common knowledge that weight loss generally becomes more challenging once you reach a specific age. Why does that happen? How can intermittent fasting help solve the problem? Can intermittent fasting help achieve healthy weight loss? Can you slow aging with this dieting method? These are a few questions you will find concise answers to in this book.

It contains up-to-date information compared to many other books on the market. It is written in simple and straightforward language to ease understanding. It breaks down the most complex terms to make for fluid assimilation. What sets it apart from other books is that it contains practical, hands-on instructions and techniques you can instantly incorporate into your daily routine.

With this book, you can start your intermittent fasting journey with confidence, knowing you have a practical and reliable guide to achieve your weight loss goals.

Chapter 1: Why Dieting Isn't Easy Over 50

"Why am I gaining weight without making changes to my dieting or exercise routine?"

The above is a question that women in their 50s often have to ask their doctors. Gaining weight without eating more or exercising less can be heartbreaking for anybody, but women are more likely to be affected.

As a woman in your 50s, you want to look as good and fit as you always have. You don't expect your age to affect anything. But to your dismay, it is affecting everything. You are gaining more weight than you want. And even though you are exercising and doing all you can to lose the extra fat, it seems like your efforts are futile.

The scenario painted above is something that anyone, men or women, over 50 can relate to, regardless of background differences. Losing weight becomes harder for most people once they reach a certain age. Aging comes with many things that cumulate to significantly inhibit weight loss, enough for you to observe that changes are happening within your body.

Suppose you have been dieting and exercising without seeing expected results. There, it means that your body is experiencing age-related changes, which may be sabotaging your efforts. As you age, you lose lean muscle mass. This results in a slower metabolism. Understandably, your physical activity also decreases, leading to reduced calorie burning.

Even if you are a fit person, you are bound to experience these alterations between the ages of 40 and 50. That is when you notice the weight gain creeping in on you gradually. You might have lost weight by cutting out a snack from your diet. But now, doing that changes nothing.

The older you get, the less your body responds to weight loss efforts. A review by the Agency for Healthcare Research and Quality explains that people gain 1 to 2 pounds every year as they age. At first, you may think this isn't much, but the result is significant weight gain over time. In a few cases, it may even lead to obesity.

Not everyone adds pounds to the point where they become overweight. Genetic makeup, physical activity level, and dietary choices are a few things that influence body weight. Still, everyone struggles with weight loss or maintenance as they get older. The difference lies in how much weight you gain.

Before we go deep into the different reasons why older people, especially women, find it harder to lose or maintain weight, I want to address a common misconception. The misconception is that men lose weight faster than women and are not affected by the age-related issues in their fifties, which is misleading.

Men, like women, also experience difficulty with weight loss and maintenance the older they get. People commonly believe that men have an advantage over women in matters of weight loss. Well, this is somewhat true, but there is a catch.

Men burn more calories than body fat because they have more lean muscle tissue than women. So, even when a man is resting and not indulging in any physical activity, he can lose weight. And when a man and a woman cut the same amounts of calories from their diets, the man still loses more weight.

It is why many people believe that men have an advantage over women. But this doesn't work out in the long run. Over the long term, both genders get an equal playing field. The main difference is that men do not undergo the same hormonal changes as women do.

When you reach the menopausal age range, estrogen production reduces to a considerable extent. The sudden decrease in estrogen levels results in transferring fat to your midsection, which consequentially increases the risk of stroke, type 2 diabetes, heart disease, and other conditions.

As a woman in your 50s, there are several reasons you might find it difficult to lose or maintain your weight.

The first reason is due to losing muscle due to age. After the age of 30, your lean muscle mass naturally declines by up to 8 percent per decade. According to a publication in the Current Opinion in Clinical Nutrition and Metabolic Care, researchers call this process sarcopenia.

Age-related conditions such as arthritis often result in reduced physical activity, which, in turn, leads to muscle loss. Another possible cause of muscle loss is prolonged injury. Individually, none of these causes significant muscle loss. But together, they make a substantial impact.

Now, you might be wondering what this has to do with you exercising, dieting, and losing weight. Well, lean muscle puts more calories to work than fat. Unless you regularly engage in strength-based exercises to build and maintain your muscles, your body will require fewer calories daily. That makes you more likely to gain weight if you keep consuming the same number of calories you did when you were younger.

Most women don't realize this, so they don't bother adjusting the calories in their diets. They continue eating the usual amount, but they find it difficult to burn calories with muscle loss. Combine this with reduced physical activities, and you have several pounds gained over time.

Another reason you may find weight loss in your 50s difficult is because of hormonal changes. As a woman, you experience specific changes that are normal and natural. Even men undergo these changes as well but in different ways. It is a part of the aging process. It explains why the Center for Disease Control's scientific data shows that middle age is the prime time for weight gain.

Menopause triggers a significant drop in your estrogen levels when you are between 45 and 55. It allows you to gain extra pounds around your belly area. Usually, the shift in fat location makes your weight gain more noticeable. It also increases your risk of developing heart disease, high cholesterol, high blood pressure, and type 2 diabetes.

And there is something called *perimenopause,* the period leading up to menopausal age. During this period, you might experience mood fluctuations, making it challenging to conform to healthy eating and exercise. Due to this, you may gain about five pounds during the transition from perimenopause to menopause.

In contrast, men start experiencing a dip in testosterone levels around 40 years old. This happens at a rate of about 1 to 2 percent every year. Testosterone in men is responsible for muscle strength, muscle mass, and fat distribution regulation. A decline in its production naturally affects all of these functions, reducing the body's effectiveness at burning calories.

Also, the growth hormone (GH) production reduces in both men and women, which further affects the body. Among other things, the growth hormone's function is to build muscle mass. It is also responsible for maintenance. So, the more it declines, the harder your body finds it to develop and maintain muscle mass. Inadvertently, this impacts the number of calories your body can effectively burn.

You accumulate more fat, build less lean muscle mass, burn fewer calories, and this continues over time. It keeps adding up, resulting in a snowball effect for your weight loss and maintenance journey.

Because of the decline in muscle mass building and maintenance, metabolism becomes slower than ever. That is another likely reason losing weight at your older age seems almost impossible. As you may already know, metabolism is a complex process that converts calories into energy inside your body.

When you have less muscle and more fat, your body burns calories slower. Remember that exercise is one way your body boosts metabolism. So, as you become less physically active at this age, your metabolism automatically becomes slower than before.

Your age isn't the only thing that impacts your metabolic rate. Sex and body size play vital roles, too. Some health conditions may also affect your metabolism. An example of such a condition is hypothyroidism.

By the time you are in your late forties and early fifties, you are likely at the peak of your career. While this is great, it poses significant weight loss challenges to you. To begin with, you may be moving less than you did when you were younger.

Maybe you spend an hour commuting to and from work and then spend up to eight hours seated at a desk every day, except weekends. You may also have a lot on your plate to where you can't spare enough time for a brisk walk or workout during the week.

To take it further, you may find you are too busy to take a lunch break most days, increasing your chances of getting calorie-condensed food from the vending machine. Ultimately, you may become subject to increased work-related stress. A study by Jen-Chieh Chuang and Jeffrey M. Zigman on Ghrelin's Roles in Stress, Mood, and Anxiety Regulation published in the International Journal of Peptides in 2010 suggests that work-related stress increases ghrelin production levels and that can make you hungrier.

Women experience significant life changes between the ages of 40 and 50, resulting in weight gain. Sometimes, you gain weight because of what is going on in your life, not the things happening within your body.

One of the most significant changes you may experience in your thirties is the start of a family. When you have a new family, the hours you spend at the gym may suddenly seem like they are more productive if you invest them in your toddler.

And you even have to engage in several parenting activities such as going on playdates, getting the homework done, and many other activities that require your undivided attention. It may seem like you don't have time for yourself anymore. Due to this, your diet and exercise routine might slip, causing you to add a few pounds.

As you have likely noticed, this chapter is merely to give you a deep insight into why weight loss isn't easy for women like you. The next chapter will reveal the basics of intermittent fasting. More important, you will discover how it can serve as your solution to these age-related issues that hinder your fitness journey.

So, let's get right to it!

Chapter 2: How Does Intermittent Fasting Work?

First, intermittent fasting is not a fad. You may find this unbelievable considering how trendy it has been for the past few years, but it is more than just another trend. Researchers and scientists have been studying this dieting strategy in laboratories around the world. Nobody invests valuable resources in what they believe to be a fad. Therefore, the first perception you should have of IF is that it is real, and it works.

Intermittent fasting is a dieting strategy that involves restricting "when" you eat to cut down your calorie intake. Unlike other dieting strategies, intermittent fasting has little to do with what you eat. Contrary to assumptions, it doesn't mean you have to starve yourself to lose weight. It doesn't give you a pass to consume as many unhealthy foods as you want, either.

The basis is that you eat within specific windows of time instead of eating different meals and snacks throughout the day. You may also call it periodic eating.

Unlike actual fasting, where you consume no meals or snacks within a specified period, intermittent fasting allows you to eat to an extent. It focuses on when to eat rather than what to eat.

Not consuming any calories for a specified number of hours per day or week can help your body burn fat more quickly and efficiently. Scientific studies suggest there are certain health benefits you can gain from fasting. An excellent example is a study titled *"Effect of Intermittent Fasting on Health, Aging, and* Disease" by De Cabo R and Mattson MP, published in the England Journal of Medicine in 2019. Calorie and mealtime restrictions can help with weight loss. But that is not all – it also reduces the risk of different diseases.

Some fasting schedules require you to fast up to 18 hours each day. It all depends on the fasting schedule you choose. In your fasting window, you do not eat anything that could increase your calorie intake. Then you can consume calories during the eating window.

The best thing about the fasting window is that it is not as difficult as it sounds. It often falls at bedtime, so most people sleep for about eight of the fasting hours. Additionally, you can consume non-calorie drinks such as coffee, tea, and water, making the whole process relatively easy for the average person.

There are several ways you can try intermittent fasting. Still, the basis of all the methods is that you choose regular periods to eat and fast. For example, you might eat during a six-hour window every day and then fast for the rest of the day. You might also choose a 24-hour fasting window after which you eat for the following 24-hour period. The point is that there are varying fasting schedules. The subsequent chapter delves deeper into the plans and shows you how you can choose one that works for you.

Most Americans eat throughout their waking hours, which is a stark contrast to the intermittent fasting eating pattern. If you eat three meals a day, with snacks, and little to no exercise, it means you are running on calories every time you eat. Simply put, you are not burning fat from your fat stores. Periodic fasting changes this unhelpful pattern by prolonging the time when your body burns through consumed calories from your last meal and starts burning your fat stores.

As you will have gathered, this dieting strategy is more about when you eat than what you eat. During your fasting window, you can consume zero-calorie beverages. And during the eating window, you only need to eat normally. You don't have to change what you eat. You still have the liberty to consume your favorite regular foods.

You shouldn't binge-eat to compensate for the fasting periods. You are unlikely to achieve your weight loss goals or become healthier if you pack your eating window with all kinds of high-calorie junk.

Many people like intermittent fasting because it does not limit them from enjoying any food they want. It teaches you to be mindful of when you eat to promote better health and fitness, but it gives no restrictions on the kinds of food to eat. Just remember that you still have to eat healthy when fasting.

Intermittent fasting is ideal for you or any woman in her fifties for several reasons. The main reason is that the limited eating window naturally limits the calories you consume every day. The previous chapter stated that weight loss becomes a challenge in the fifties because women continue to consume the same number of calories they did at a younger age. Still, the body finds them harder to burn.

When you start fasting, your calorie intake automatically reduces, which means that your body has fewer calories to burn. The fewer calories consumed, the easier the body can burn fat.

The benefits of intermittent fasting are not limited to calorie restriction, particularly for older women. Many experts disagree with those who believe that IF works only because it limits food intake. These experts believe that the results people get from periodic fasting are much better than general meal schedules that involve consuming the same number of calories and other nutrients.

Some experts also suggest that daily food abstinence for several hours does not just restrict calorie consumption – it does more than that. Time-restricted fasting causes specific metabolic changes in the body. These changes account for some of its synergistic benefits.

The three changes are:

- **Insulin:** During your fasting window, insulin levels drop to encourage fat burning.

- **HGH**: As insulin levels drop, your HGH levels rise to improve muscle growth and fat burning.

- **Noradrenaline:** In response to fasting, your nervous system releases noradrenaline to your cells to inform them they need to burn fat for fuel

These changes cumulate to cause "metabolic switching," which scientists believe to be responsible for intermittent fasting benefits. Metabolic switching is simply when your body depletes its glycogen supply within 10 to 12 hours of fasting, after which it burns ketones. That is a sort of fuel that your liver makes from stored fat.

The switch from glycogen to ketones affects other chemicals in your body and your immune signals and growth factors. But ketones are not the only thing that happens. The periodic fasting and eating windows also activate genes and signaling pathways, making your neurons stronger.

Before we go deep into how intermittent fasting may be beneficial specifically to women in their 50s, here are a few evidence-based advantages according to science.

1. Changes in Cells, Genes, and Hormones Functions

One of the scientifically proven advantages of intermittent fasting is that it changes how your cells, genes, and hormones function. Several things happen in the body during the fasting window. For one, your body triggers some vital cellular repair processes. It also changes your hormone levels to make your body fat storage more accessible.

Insulin levels drop significantly, initiating the fat-burning process. The growth hormone production also increases as much as five-fold. As noted previously, increment in the production of this hormone facilitates muscle gain and fat burning. There are tons of other health benefits.

When you put off eating for a while, your body also repairs your cells. For example, it naturally removes waste materials from your cellular organs. Changes further occur through gene expression. Some changes contribute to protection against disease and longevity.

Most benefits associated with intermittent fasting result from hormones, cell functions, and gene expression changes.

2. Burns Belly Fat

The midsection is possibly the one place where women find it hardest to burn fat. Even in your twenties and thirties, losing belly fat is hard enough. But when you become older, it becomes even more challenging. Intermittent fasting can make it easy for you because it makes you eat fewer meals and snacks. Most people that try intermittent fasting end up taking in fewer calories unless they eat much more than they should during their eating windows.

The changes in hormone function resulting from fasting facilitate the foundation for fat burning and weight loss. Reduced insulin levels, increased growth hormone production, and higher noradrenaline levels all enhance the body's ability to break fat down, facilitating an opening to convert to energy.

Due to this, periodic fasting accelerates your metabolic rate by up to 14 percent, helping you burn even more calories than you usually do. Intermittent fasting helps on both sides of the calorie equation. It increases your metabolic rate and therefore boosts calorie-burning. It also reduces food intake and, thus, decreases calorie consumption.

Based on a review of the scientific literature, you can lose up to 8 percent of your weight over 24 weeks by fasting intermittently. This is a substantial amount of weight loss. Since metabolism generally slows as a person ages, intermittent fasting is key to increasing your metabolic rate and burning as many calories as you want.

The review further shows that intermittent fasting ensures less muscle loss than other calorie restriction methods. This means it can help reduce the loss of muscle that occurs to women in their fifties.

Considering all of these, you can tell that intermittent fasting is a powerful weight loss technique.

3. Reduces Type 2 Diabetes Risk

Intermittent fasting has been proven to reduce insulin resistance, which lowers your risk of developing type 2 diabetes. In the last few decades, type 2 diabetes has become common among Americans. Higher blood sugar levels are the highlight in the context of insulin resistance.

Anything that can help you reduce insulin resistance will inadvertently lower blood sugar levels and lower type 2 diabetes risk. Not surprisingly, the study mentioned earlier also shows that intermittent fasting is incredibly beneficial to improving insulin resistance and lowering blood sugar levels. The evidence shows that the benefits are impressive.

Through fasting, up to six percent of blood sugar levels are reduced, while insulin is reduced by up to thirty-one percent. So, if you at risk of developing the condition, intermittent fasting can do much more than help you burn fat.

4. De-Escalates Stress and Inflammation

Oxidative stress contributes to aging and different chronic diseases. It is triggered when free radicals, which are unstable molecules in the body, react with other vital molecules, resulting in damage. Several studies on the benefits of intermittent fasting have shown that it can boost the body's ability to resist oxidative stress.

Besides, the studies also show that intermittent fasting helps in the fight against inflammation. Medically inclined people know that inflammation is the number one driver of all kinds of common diseases.

Oxidative stress and inflammation tend to affect older people more than younger ones. Fasting periodically is a proven way to protect yourself against the aging process and improve your body's immunity against diseases.

5. Improves Heart Health

All over the world, heart disease is recognized as the most significant cause of death. There are various factors associated with the risk of heart disease. Evidence suggests that intermittent fasting improves these health markers. Some of them include blood pressure, blood sugar levels, inflammatory markers, LDL cholesterol, and blood triglycerides.

Most of the evidence comes from research done on animals. Further studies need to be done on the effect of heart disease in humans. But even the potential is exciting.

6. Autophagy

When you fast, your body triggers something known as autophagy. It is the process through which your body gets rid of waste from the cells. It involves your cells breaking down and metabolizing any dysfunctional and broken proteins built up in the cells over time. When this happens, your protection against diseases such as cancer and Alzheimer's disease increases.

Other benefits of intermittent fasting include:

- Improvement of physical performance
- Enhanced thinking and memory abilities
- Prevention of diabetes and obesity
- Decreased tissue damage

You are probably curious about how intermittent fasting can enhance your body's ability to burn calories and fat.

As explained earlier, decreased metabolism is one of the affective factors for challenging weight loss in older women. Most women are aware of this. When metabolism slows down, you find it harder to burn calories, which makes you add more pounds. With intermittent fasting, you can cut down the calories you consume to shed excess weight or even keep it off.

On average, a woman needs to cut at least 100 calories from her daily diet. Once you are in your 50s, the first step should be to cut your calorie intake from 1,800 daily to 1,600 per day. If you keep consuming 1,800 calories, you may add up to 10 pounds every year.

Intermittent fasting can help you cut down your calorie intake so you don't consume more than your body can effectively burn. You might like using IF to reduce calorie intake because you don't have to deprive yourself of certain foods. You can still eat what you want, but if specific foods add more calories than necessary to your diet, giving them up will help your journey.

Another problem mentioned in chapter one was reduced physical activity. How can intermittent fasting help with that? Well, it would be illogical to say that fasting can completely replace exercise and physical activity, but it can contribute.

Like fasting, exercise also triggers autophagy because it is key to cell regeneration. It does more than that, though. Autophagy helps to cleanse the body to optimize it, making fat-burning easier than ever. This process ensues in many benefits for you. Among these are building insulin resistance and slowing the aging process. Without autophagy, you may become prone to weight gain, higher cholesterol, and impaired brain function.

Autophagy is triggered by positive stress, which you get from exercising and engaging in tasking physical activities. Skipping meals is another way you can cause positive stress and, ultimately, initiate your body's autophagy process.

So, even if your activities are reduced due to age, fasting periodically can serve the same purpose. But fasting cannot serve as a total replacement for exercise. You still need to work out. Exercising has tons of other benefits that you cannot get from fasting. The best thing is to combine both to get the best result.

Activities such as walking, jogging, and swimming are easy on the lower back and knees, making them ideal for older people. Both are also effective for jump-starting metabolism and burning calories. We'll discuss this more in a subsequent chapter.

Sarcopenia, as you have learned, is the loss of muscle mass. It is a natural side-effect of the aging process. Intermittent fasting can be useful to combat muscle loss in less active adults. Age-induced muscle loss may be inevitable, but it's manageable if approached in the right way.

Without exercise or intense physical activity, weight loss typically occurs due to losing lean mass and fat mass. Your muscles are a part of your lean mass. Everything in your body, except fat, is part of your lean mass.

When you try any diet targeted at weight loss, you are likely to lose your lean mass. That shows that dieting methods, including intermittent fasting, may cause loss of muscle mass. Some studies have shown that intermittent fasting causes one to lose up to 2 pounds of lean mass, but other studies showed contrasting results.

This has led many researchers to suggest that intermittent fasting likely affects lean mass maintenance during weight loss more than other non-fasting diets. Although extensive research has not been done on this, it does show that the effect can vary from person to person.

Overall, the consensus is that periodic fasting does not cause more muscle loss than other types of diets. If you combine mild exercises with intermittent fasting, you can successfully reduce the rate of muscle mass loss. Intermittent fasting cannot be used to gain muscle. But if done the right way, it's used to reduce the loss.

Strength-training exercises are the best way to reduce the consistent loss of muscle in your older age. Doing pushups a few times a week while fasting intermittently can make all the difference you want in your weight loss journey. Note that strength-training may also prevent bone loss, another primary concern for any woman in her fifties.

There are several ways intermittent fasting counters the issues that could make weight loss more difficult for you in your older years. These are just a few of the important ones you should know.

Ultimately, the most exciting benefit of this dieting strategy is that it could potentially extend your lifespan. In other words, it can help boost longevity for its practitioners. Studies done on rats suggest that IF improves longevity as continuous calorie restriction does.

Several results of the studies conducted were dramatic. One study showed that rats that fasted periodically lived up to 83% longer than those that didn't fast.

While this study has not been replicated with humans, it confirms that IF may have anti-aging benefits for older people.

Considering the many known benefits due to metabolic switching and other health markers, intermittent fasting will help you do much more than lose weight. It can affect the quality of your health and life. Automatically reducing your calorie intake can help you lose weight and live a healthier and longer life.

Healthy eating is simple, but it is also challenging to maintain. One of the many obstacles is that you have to put in maximum effort to plan and cook healthy meals. Intermittent fasting is your key to easy dieting because it does not require you to prepare, cook, and clean up as many meals as you did before.

For this very reason, its popularity among fitness and weight enthusiast continues to grow. By incorporating it into your everyday dieting routine, you can lose weight and improve your health while living a simple life simultaneously.

Throughout the remaining chapters, you will discover more about why intermittent fasting has become a popular trend among life-hackers. Read on.

Chapter 3: Types of Intermittent Fasting Plans

Depending on your lifestyle and weight loss goals, there are several patterns of fasting to follow. Individually, every single method is effective, but if you don't figure out which one is more suitable for you, the results may not be as impressive as you want.

The difference in intermittent fasting methods lies in the calorie allowances and the number of fasting hours. The experience you get from this dieting method is affected wholly by you. There are seven ways you can fast intermittently. To help decide which is more appropriate, this chapter unravels the science and research behind each type of fasting and, more importantly, how you can maintain the diet you choose.

The 12:12 Plan

This is an intermittent fasting pattern where you fast for 12 hours and eat for the other 12 hours every day. For beginners, the 12:12 plan is one of the easiest methods to start with. It requires you to restrict your daily food and calorie intake to within a 12-hour eating window rather than eating throughout the day.

Once your 12-hour eating window is gone, you are not advised to consume anything that might give your body calories. Your options are limited to zero-calorie drinks like water and black coffee. Fasting for just 12 hours every day is all you need to reap the fantastic benefits of this dieting strategy.

The rules for this method are simple. You need to choose a 12-hour fasting window you can adhere to every day for as long as you plan to fast. This plan has a relatively small fasting window, which typically falls into sleep time. You can consume a specific number of calories each day without having to worry about burning fat.

The easiest way you can follow this plan is to make sure that your sleep time is included in your fasting window. For example, you may fast between 8 p.m. and 8 a.m. To adhere to this timeframe, you would have to finish dinner every day before 8 p.m. and wait until 7 a.m. before you can eat another meal. Naturally, you would be asleep for much of the time between your eating and fasting window.

Fasting for 12 hours is the lowest you can do, as that is when your body can trigger metabolic switching to burn fat for fuel. After you become familiar with fasting and the feeling within your body, you can swiftly change from this beginner plan to a more advanced one.

The longer the hours in your fasting window, the more fat your body can burn after metabolic switching occurs.

The 16:8 Plan

This particular method is one of the most popular plans among intermittent fasting enthusiasts. Some even believe it to be the most effective. The 16:8 plan involves fasting every day for 16 hours while limiting your eating window to 8 hours. Even though the eating window may look relatively small, you can still fit in two to three meals within your eating window. Martin Berkhan, a fitness expert, popularized the 16:8 plan, and several people call it the Lean Gains Protocol.

16:8 intermittent fasting pattern works by supporting your body's circadian rhythm, which you may also call its internal clock. Following this plan means you abstain from food at night and part of the morning and afternoon. The eating period tends to start at midday.

As with other types of IF patterns, you have no restrictions on the types of foods you can eat during the eating window. There are also no restrictions on the amount of food to eat. Still, you are generally advised to consume the same amount you usually do during mealtime. The flexibility of this method explains why most people find it relatively easy to follow.

The simplest way to follow this plan is to choose a fasting window that includes the time you sleep. Some IF experts suggest that fasters should finish all food intake in the early evening, possibly around 6 to 7 p.m. Metabolism typically slows down after early evening, although this approach may not be feasible for everyone.

Your daily routine may make it impossible for you to consume your evening meal until later. You need to avoid food for at least 2 hours before your bedtime. Below are a few 8-hour eating windows from which you can choose:

- 9 a.m. to 5 p.m.
- Noon to 8 p.m.
- 10 a.m. to 6 p.m.

Within these timeframes, you can eat and snack conveniently. Regular healthy eating is vital to prevent peaks and dips in blood sugar levels and to reduce the possibility of excessive hunger. If you have to, don't be afraid to experiment with different timeframes to figure out the best eating and fasting window for your lifestyle.

To maximize the potential benefits of the 16:8 diet, you must stick to nutritious foods and beverages during your eating period. Don't see fasting as an opportunity to consume as many junk foods as possible. Fill up your diet with nutrient-rich foods to round it out and gain the benefits of periodic fasting.

Although it has many health benefits, restricting yourself to an 8-hour window has drawbacks, and this means it may not be right for you. The restriction on food intake can push you to eat more than usual during your eating window. Subconsciously try to make up for hours expended on fasting without realizing it.

Rather than help you shed extra pounds, this may cause more weight gain, digestive problems and even cause you to develop unhealthy eating habits. Suppose you don't choose a timeframe that fits right into your daily routine. There, this fasting plan may also cause adverse short-term effects such as fatigue, hunger, and weakness. These typically subside once your body gets more familiar with the new routine.

The 5:2 Plan

Also called the fast diet, this plan is the most popular intermittent fasting method according to current trends. Michael Mosley, a British journalist, is responsible for popularizing the 5:2 technique. The name derives from the fasting pattern involving eating for five days of the week and fasting for the remaining two days.

You need not fast for two entire days. The idea is to restrict calorie intake to just 1200 calories on both days. This means you must not consume over 600 calories per day. Even though this method may seem like a lot, most people agree that it is easier to stick to than any other calorie-restricted diet.

Typically, you can eat for your 5-day eating window without restricting yourself to any specific amounts of calories. Then, within the two-day fasting window, you have to cut your calorie intake to a quarter of your daily calorie needs; you consume only 500 to 600 calories per day.

This plan allows you to choose whichever days of the week you prefer for fasting. You need to make sure there is one non-fasting day between. One typical pattern of following this plan is to make Monday and Thursday your fasting days, while the rest of the week will be non-fasting. Eat two to three small meals on every fasting day, then eat normally for the remainder of the week.

Again, eating "normally" does not mean you get to eat anything you want. You are discouraged from binge-eating junk foods as this can jeopardize your whole routine. You may gain weight instead of shedding it. Eat the same amount of food as you usually would if you weren't fasting at all.

If done the right way, the 5:2 diet can prove highly useful for weight loss. It helps you consume fewer calories per week, which enhances your body's metabolic rate. There is no definitive way to eat during the five-day fasting window. But there are approaches you can take.

For example, some people can't get their body moving without a small breakfast to jump-start the day. For others, starting the day with breakfast is a sure way to boost hunger throughout their day. People like that need to wait if they can before their first meal of the day.

Thus, this fasting method's meal plan may vary from person to person, although only slightly. On fast days, your schedules may include either of:

- Three small meals, which include an early breakfast, lunch, and late dinner
- Early afternoon meal and late-night dinner
- A brief breakfast and lunch, without dinner
- A single meal of breakfast or dinner

You can pick any of these schedules or change them from week to week. That decision is yours to make. The point is to drastically cut down the number of calories you consume. If you consume 1,800 calories on an average day, only consume 450 calories during your fasting window. If your daily calorie intake is usually 2,000, then reduce it to 500 calories on fast days.

If you do a lot of endurance exercise, don't fast on days when you work out. Consult with your doctor to make sure this fasting plan is compatible with any other physical activity you regularly engage in. Evaluate your training plan to make sure it aligns with the dieting plan.

Eat Stop Eat

This approach is one of the easiest you can take when it comes to intermittent fasting. As a beginner, if you cannot do the 12:12 method, you can begin your journey with this one. Brad Pilon, an intermittent fasting expert, is the originator of this method. Pilon researched short-term fasting and its benefits, and the findings were used to come up with the Eat Stop Eat fasting style.

According to Pilon, the best way to lose the extra pounds in your body is by fasting for 24 hours at least once or twice per week. During the non-fasting days, you can eat normally. But you are not to consume any calorie-containing food during your fasting window or days. By doing this, you can create a calorie deficit in your body, which will, over time, lead to effective weight loss.

For instance, if you typically consume 1800 calories daily, the Eat Stop Eat method two days a week will cause a calorie deficit of 3600 each week. To lose a pound of fat, you need a deficit of 3500 calories. Thus, you can potentially lose more than a pound every week if you follow this dieting style.

This method is not a fluke. A simple search on Google will bring up tons of positive reviews from people who have successfully used it to shed extra pounds. If done the right way, you can use Eat Stop Eat to lose up to 9 pounds in a month. That, of course, depends on your body, but using this approach will help you shed a couple of pounds.

As a newbie to the whole fasting thing, following this method is recommended because you do not have to fast every day. This means you don't have to worry about the fasting routine affecting your regular day-to-day schedule. You also have the freedom to decide when your fasting days are, which makes it easy to choose whenever is convenient for you.

For example, suppose weekend days allow you to engage in activities that can distract you from cravings. There, you can simply choose the weekend for your fasting window.

This diet is similar to the 5:2 plan, so many beginners confuse them, but there is a vital difference between both fasting styles. The 5:2 diet restricts your calorie intake on fasting days to 500. The Eat Stop Eat diet restricts you from calorie intake for 24 hours. During the fasting window, you may not consume any food or drink that contains calories.

Not eating for 24 hours might seem like a difficult task, and rightfully so. But with the 5:2 diet, the 500 calories intake can trigger hunger and facilitate physical discomfort. On the other hand, eating nothing within a 24-hour window helps suppress your appetite until your window elapses and ready for food consumption.

There is no specific drawback to using this style of fasting. But know that most of the scientific studies done on intermittent fasting have focused on the 16:8 and Alternate Day Fasting methods. Therefore, one cannot give science-backed evidence of any drawback.

Still, that does not imply that this approach is ineffective or has fewer advantages than other fasting methods. The only apparent drawback is that some people may find it difficult to fast for 24 hours without food intake. Consequentially, they may end up overeating when the eating window begins.

Any newbie to fasting is more likely to experience this slight problem. Nevertheless, once the body adapts to the new state of metabolism and energy balance, this problem will cease to exist. This fasting method is not appropriate for pregnant women, diabetics, or anyone with an eating disorder. Before you get started with Eat Stop Eat, learn your needs, goals, and fasting ability.

Alternate Day Fasting

Alternate day fasting (ADF) is relatively straightforward. It is an approach to intermittent fasting that involves fasting every other day. It has several versions of itself, but the end goal of all the versions is to help you cut down the intake of calories. One standard version of ADF is called modified fasting, which encourages you to consume 25% of your daily calorie intake on fasting days.

Basically, you fast on one day, eat what you want the next day, fast the following day again, and continue like that until you complete your fasting cycle. This way, you just need to limit what you eat half of the week. During the fasting window, you can consume as many calorie-devoid beverages and drinks as you desire.

The most common version of ADF is "The Every Other Day Diet." This version was popularized by Dr. Krista Vardy, who is also the researcher with the most studies done on ADF. Whether you consume the calories at lunch or dinner, the weight loss benefits remain the same. You may also consume small meals throughout the day if you don't go beyond the specified number of calories.

Depending on your body and needs, alternate-day fasting may prove easier for you than other types of intermittent fasting. A study on the effect of alternate-day fasting on weight loss among obese adults found this method is not necessarily superior to daily calorie restriction. Most of the ADF studies focus on the modified version, which allows you to consume 500 calories on fasting days. Some experts believe this is more sustainable than the full fasts.

It is impossible to pinpoint the specific effects of ADF on hunger. Depending on the individual, hunger may reduce on fasting days or remain unchanged. But the consensus is that calorie-restrictive fasting is much more convenient than full fasts.

All weight loss methods seem to trigger a drop in the body's resting metabolic rate. This happens when the body induces starvation mode. Technically, the process is called adaptive thermogenesis. It often occurs when an individual severely restricts their calorie intake.

When strict calorie restriction happens, the body automatically starts conserving energy by decreasing the calories it burns daily. This, inadvertently, causes weight loss to stop. Understandably, an experience like this can make you feel miserable. Fortunately, ADF does not appear to cause a dip in the body's metabolic rate, based on research.

Spontaneous Meal Skipping

This is an unstructured intermittent fasting plan that allows you to simply skip meals occasionally. For example, you may skip a meal when you don't feel hungry or don't have time to cook or eat.

There is a popular misconception that people have to eat every few hours to avoid losing muscle or going into starvation mode. Your body was designed to effectively handle prolonged hunger. So, missing a meal occasionally won't affect you in any way. It will help you lose or maintain your weight.

Thus, if you don't feel hungry on certain days, you can take advantage of that to skip breakfast or lunch and have a healthy dinner. Or, if you are traveling and can't get food anywhere, use that time to practice spontaneous meal skipping.

The method may not be as effective as other plans like 5:2 or 16:8, but it has its advantages. Just eat healthy meals during your eating window.

Warrior Diet

The warrior diet was created by Ori Hofmekler, an ex-member of the Israeli Special Forces, who became a fitness and nutrition expert. The diet is a type of intermittent fasting which is founded on ancient eating patterns followed by warriors. It involves eating very little during the day and then overeating at night.

Hofmekler says it is meant to "improve the way we eat, feel, perform, and look" by triggering stress in the body via reduced calorie intake. The result is to trigger the human "survival instincts."

This diet is not based on any science. It was designed purely on Hofmekler's personal beliefs and observations. To follow this diet, you have to under-eat for at least 20 hours of the day, then overeat as much food as you can at night.

During the fasting window, you are encouraged to eat vegetables, raw fruit, hard-boiled eggs, other dairy products in small amounts, and zero-calorie drinks. After the 20-hour window has passed, you can binge-eat whatever you want within the 4-hour eating window. But you are encouraged to stick to healthy, organic foods.

To start the warrior diet, you are urged to stick to a three-week plan segmented into different phases. The three-phase plan's basis is to enhance your body's ability to use fat as fuel or energy. The first phase in week one is for detox. Week two is called the "High fat" phase. The final phase is the "Concluding fat loss" stage.

Each phase encourages you to consume unprocessed, organic foods, but you still have the liberty of choosing what you eat. The last stage mostly cycles between the high carb and high protein intake. Once all three phases are completed, you are to begin all over again. But rather than go through the complete cycle, you may forgo the first two phases and simply adhere to the general guidelines.

The guidelines include consuming low-calorie foods and drinks for 20 hours and then consuming protein-rich, organic meals during your feasting phase.

The warrior diet has several limitations that make it inappropriate for most people. The 4-hour eating window makes it highly unsustainable for many people. It leaves little room for dieters to participate in regular social activities such as having lunch or breakfast with friends.

But this does not apply to everyone. Some people are not necessarily affected when they consume a few calories over the fasting period. You may experiment to determine if this pattern of eating is ideal for your lifestyle.

The warrior diet is inappropriate for any of the people below:

- Pregnant women
- Nursing mothers
- Children
- Athletes
- Those with eating disorders
- Underweight people
- Individuals with cancer, heart failure, type 1 diabetes, and other conditions

Some women may follow this diet with zero adverse effects. In contrast, others need to stay off it because of its impact on hormones. Common side effects include anxiety, insomnia, fluctuating periods, and other health disturbances.

Picking an intermittent fasting plan well suited to your lifestyle is crucial. You can experiment with a few strategies discussed to determine which is more appropriate for you. If you so wish, you can even change the pattern you use occasionally. Just don't do it too often.

As impressive as time-restricted eating is, it simply isn't for everyone. In the next chapter, you will discover if it is for you or not. Who can practice intermittent fasting and who can't? Let's learn more!

Chapter 4: Who Should and Who Should Not Fast

Fasting may be a useful weight-loss hack, but it certainly isn't for everyone. In pursuing health, intermittent fasting can be misused. Any diet that involves time-restricted eating for extended periods is most definitely not suitable for certain people. Several factors determine who should fast and who should not. It is best to know if fasting is safe for you before incorporating it into your daily routine.

If you are healthy and hydrated, fasting shouldn't be harmful to you. If you have health conditions, it may be bad for you. Typically, your body requires minerals, vitamins, and other nutrients to stay healthy.

Foods are your number one source of these nutritional requirements. Without getting enough, you could develop symptoms such as dizziness, fatigue, dehydration, and constipation. You may also find it difficult to withstand colder temperatures. For the wrong person, fasting can be life-threatening.

As long as you are healthy and fit with no diagnosed conditions that could jeopardize your health, you can fast. But if you have one or more of the following conditions, you shouldn't try intermittent fasting.

Diabetes

Diabetic individuals suffer frequent spikes and drops in their blood sugar levels throughout the day. The last thing they require is for fasting to heighten the fluctuation in their blood glucose responses.

Those with type 1 diabetes are especially cautioned to stay away from fasting because their pancreas cannot produce insulin, which is the hormone responsible for transferring sugar from the bloodstream to the body's different cells.

Individuals with type 1 diabetes need insulin injections to avoid inducing a state of hyperglycemia, which is when there is excess sugar in the bloodstream. If you are diabetic and on medication for insulin, you need to consult your doctor before intermittent fasting.

Fasting while you are on diabetes medications can cause a dangerous low in your blood sugar. But if your doctor gives the go-ahead, you will need close monitoring to continue with fasting. Anyone with low blood sugar should avoid intermittent fasting because consuming food every day is crucial to maintaining sufficient blood sugar levels.

Pregnancy or Breastfeeding

Fasting during pregnancy or while breastfeeding is a threat to child development. So, pregnant and breastfeeding women are not encouraged to engage in intermittent fasting because they have high caloric needs.

During pregnancy, a woman has to consume specific calories to aid milk production and fetal development. While no study has suggested that fasting can inhibit fetal growth, it is best to be on the safer side by fulfilling the daily calorie requirements. Fasting interferes with caloric intake, so the ideal thing is to stay away from it during pregnancy.

Even if you aren't pregnant, fasting may still not be ideal for anyone trying to get pregnant. Experts suggest that intermittent fasting may cause fertility issues and changes in menstruation due to hormonal effects. It also disrupts metabolism and may even prompt early menopause in women who are yet in their fifties.

Eating Disorders

The Academy of Nutrition and Dietetics says that disordered eating "is used to describe a range of irregular eating behaviors that may or may not warrant a diagnosis of a specific eating disorder."

Eating disorders are not described as a diagnosis. Instead, they are treated as a descriptive phase. Suppose one doesn't address irregular eating habits or patterns. In that case, it may turn into actual eating disorders such as bulimia nervosa, anorexia nervosa, or binge eating.

If you have ever experienced any irregular eating pattern or have an eating disorder, it is best to steer clear of intermittent fasting or any other type of fasting. Any diet that encourages restricting calorie intake can trigger a disorder in people with a history of irregular eating patterns. For everyone, but someone with a history, in particular, listening to your body is crucial.

You must be mindful of what makes you feel physical, mentally, and emotionally well. If time-restricted eating does not make you feel adequate, it means that intermittent fasting is not the right diet for you.

Sleep Problems

Getting enough sleep at night isn't a choice. Adequate sleep every night is a necessity. It is key to repairing and healing your muscles. Sleep supports brain function and maintains your emotional well-being.

Going to bed on an empty stomach can make it hard for your body to relax and sleep. Fasting makes the brain stay on alert, which inadvertently causes your body to be restless. If the end of your eating window is early in the day, falling asleep or staying asleep may become a struggle for you. Sleep inadequacy makes you vulnerable to a couple of health risks since sleep time is when your body can do all the healing and repairing work it is meant to do.

Additionally, blood sugar levels drop during the fasting window, and this can disrupt your sleeping pattern. You may wake abruptly during the night due to anxiety. A disrupted sleeping pattern is dangerous to your overall health. It is especially harmful if the disruption frequently happens during the most pivotal stage when the Random Eye Movement (REM) cycle occurs.

The REM stage is key to retaining vital information you learn and process during the day to commit it to memory. It happens multiple times throughout your sleep, which is why it is called a cycle. Besides these, disruptions can lead to other complications that may not immediately become apparent.

Not getting enough sleep can also interfere with weight management. If intermittent fasting causes you sleep problems, it might help you gain more weight instead of losing it.

Insufficient Muscle Mass

If you are trying to build your muscle mass, intermittent fasting may be unsafe for you. In fact, experts suggest that it is not ideal. Muscle building requires you to consume protein-rich foods several times throughout the day. This is better than jam-packing it in a single eating window.

Experts say this is because the average person's body cannot metabolize more than 35g of protein in a sitting. Suppose you want your body to metabolize properly. There, you are better off eating your protein meals at different times across your whole day. Without proper metabolization, excess protein stores as fat rather than muscle.

To build muscle, you need to spread your protein consumption through multiple meals in a day. Also, consume one protein-rich snack before bedtime. These are the two research-backed ways for you to achieve optimum muscle-building results. Narrowing your consumption window to just 8 or 12 hours is counteractive to this approach.

But if you would still like to go ahead, talk to your doctor about the safest ways to engage in intermittent fasting without countering your muscle-building effort.

Digestion Issues

Combining digestion problems with intermittent fasting can worsen their health situation. If you have any issue with digestion, you already know that they are cumbersome enough to deal with individually. Now, if you add an irregular eating schedule to the mix, you can compound the problem.

Extended periods of fasting can lead to more gastrointestinal distress. Even if you have no digestion problems, prolonged fasting can serve as a trigger. This happens because prolonged periods of fasting disrupt your digestive system's everyday activities. This results in indigestion, constipation, and bloating.

If you use an IF method that requires a prolonged fast, such as the warrior diet, you may consume one large meal at the end of your fasting window, but it can cause gastrointestinal stress. People with sensitive guts should be particularly wary of practicing any form of fasting.

Weak Immune System

Women who face a major illness or have just experienced one should not practice IF without seeking their doctor's advice first. Often, regular caloric intake is necessary to keep the immune system healthy and maintain lean muscle. It is even essential for those with a weak immune system or conditions such as cancer. It is something that you cannot compromise if you have any of both conditions.

Before you engage in fasting, speak to your doctor to make sure that your body can handle the effect. To boost your immune response, start by skipping IF from your dieting routine. There are tons of other dieting techniques safer for you to lose weight.

Besides these health reasons, many other factors may hinder your ability to fast effectively. Shown below are factors that hamper participation in intermittent fasting.

- **Lifestyle**

Intermittent fasting is not just a dieting technique; it is a lifestyle – and it must align or fit into the dieter's lifestyle. Your work schedule is part of what comprises your lifestyle. It influences your ability to make IF a part of your routine. If your work does not support the fasting hours, then there is little you can do.

For instance, if your job requires you to work the night shift, it may have a negative effect on you. Working the night shift means you sleep during the day. If you follow an IF technique with the eating window during the day, how do you work around that?

What if your fasting window falls within the time you are hard at work? Or worse, what if your schedule is inconsistent and prone to regular change? There, the fasting intervals can leave you feeling cold, give you headaches and mood swings. These side effects could make you less productive at work because they are distracting.

The ideal thing is to settle for another dieting strategy if intermittent fasting does not match your lifestyle.

• Medications

Some people are on medications with food as a prerequisite; in other words, their medications cannot be used in the absence of food. Without it, they can leave you feeling light-headed and nauseous, among many other side effects.

Prolonged fasting periods can also affect those who take supplements and vitamins daily. For example, those with anemia or low iron count in their bloodstream usually need to take iron supplements daily to maintain iron levels.

Iron supplements typically cause nausea, but the feeling can be suppressed with food. If you have a flexible schedule for taking your supplements, then fasting shouldn't be a problem, but if you have to take the medications at a specific time of the day with food, things may get a little tricky.

Ultimately, it is simply not ideal to start time-restricted eating if you are on medications that can't be administered without food intake.

• Job

Food provides energy and sustenance, which, in turn, enable you to focus. Extreme pangs of hunger make you think about food, diverting your attention from any tasks on the ground. Naturally, everyone reacts to periodic fasting differently. The side-effects generally depend on the individual doing the fasting.

In the initial stage, IF hinders everyone's ability to focus. If you have never had to go long periods without food, you will also experience this. If you have a job that requires intense focus and concentration, IF may pose a problem.

Although many people report energy increase during fasting windows, most people experience low energy levels, reduced concentration, and fatigue. These affect productivity. Suppose you have a career or regularly engage in activities that require great attention and energy. In that case, prolonged fasting may be impractical for you.

- **Intensive Training**

As you have likely assumed, combining intermittent fasting with any high-intensity activity or training cycle is not safe or ideal. You might practice intermittent fasting if you regularly engage in CrossFit or train for marathons. Usually, you will need to consume something tangible before exercising. This helps to power you through the duration of your workout.

It is also of extreme importance you eat something after you finish your workout. During an intense training exercise, you deplete your glycogen stores, and minor tears happen in your muscles. A recovery meal within two hours plus regular meals every four hours is the key to refilling our glycogen stores. It also helps to repair and rebuild the tears in your muscle throughout the rest of your day.

Skipping the post-training meal delays your recovery and eventually inhibits the build and repair of muscles, which is essential.

Whether you have any of the conditions explained above or not, you should still discuss intermittent fasting with your doctor before you begin. We all live in one big obesogenic food environment.

The U.S. is generally a toxic place because a significant percentage of the population does not engage in healthy eating habits. Even if nothing obstructs you from trying intermittent fasting, be sure that you have a robust social network to support you through your journey. This sometimes makes all the difference for dieters. With supportive friends and family members, enduring low-calorie days over the long haul should prove easy.

Chapter 5: How to Safely Lose Weight While Fasting

Losing weight after turning 50 involves more than simply fasting. You need more than diet and exercise. The key is not just to lose weight but to lose it healthily. Besides fasting, you must develop other habits crucial to boosting your overall health and wellness. These habits should be geared toward improving both your physical and mental health.

Even while fasting, there are steps you can take to shake up your whole routine. Incorporating new activities and habits into your daily schedule will enable you to lose weight healthily while improving your mental and physical wellness.

Below, you will find many of the best weight-loss habits according to expert fitness and wellness trainers and dietitians. Building up these habits and following any tips you learn in this chapter is your key to shedding pounds with intermittent fasting and ensuring they stay off your body for good.

Consult Your Doctor

The first step you should take as you begin your 50s' fitness journey is talking to your doctor. Discuss the weight loss plan you want to follow extensively to make sure it is practical for you.

Your doctor should assess your health's current state to inform you of any potential problems affecting your weight loss journey. More importantly, you should work together to create the perfect plan that includes diet, exercise, and other necessary things. If needed, your doctor may even recommend a personal trainer or physical therapist for you.

Some commonly used medications enable weight gain, so let your doctor check your prescription meds to evaluate if there are any. Trying to lose weight while on drugs that make that impossible is a futile exercise. Antidepressants, diabetes medication, and high blood pressure medications are common ones to look out for.

If you are on any of these, your healthcare provider should be able to replace them with weight-neutral medications that may even promote weight loss.

Set Realistic Weight Loss Goals

Being as realistic as possible is the key to healthy weight loss. Don't set out to lose 20 pounds in a month because not only is it unrealistic, but it is also unhealthy. Honesty is a virtue, so be honest with yourself about your needs and current state of health.

Consider how you feel. Are you as healthy as you should be? If you aren't, taking extreme weight loss measures should be last on your to-do list. Taking the step to lose weight is equal to making a huge life change, requiring mental fortitude.

You need to break down your goals into smaller, realistic ones. The more real they are, the more achievable. Focus on the little, positive changes that can make a difference in your lifestyle. Take your mind away from the number on the scale and concentrate on the things that matter. Doing that will give you the motivation you need to achieve all your goals.

The little achievements amount to the most prominent goals achieved. As the saying goes, "Triumph makes courage grow." So, the more you accomplish the small goals, the more your courage grows to make you push even further.

Do Hormone Checks

Things might get a little complicated here because most times, hormones aren't even responsible for weight gain. However, your physical examination with your doctor might show signs of hormone irregularities. If this happens, the right thing to do is to check on your hormone levels.

As you age, your body's hormone levels decline, making your body start storing fats instead of burning them. If the hormones are at abnormal levels, you may need to take steps to whip them back into shape.

This can go a long way toward helping you burn fat and lose weight. As a woman trying to get fit in your fifties, you must focus on your testosterone production. In the medical community, people tend to concentrate on the loss of estrogen in older women. Few people know testosterone sufficiency is just as important.

A study conducted at the University of Macau confirms that balance in testosterone levels promotes weight loss and shrinks belly fat by reducing blood glucose levels. So, getting your hormones checked is one way you can lose weight as healthily as possible.

Know Your Caloric Needs

Calorie needs in women vary depending on lean body mass, metabolism, size, and activity level. According to the Dietary Guidelines for Americans, the estimated caloric needs for women over 50 based on activity level are:

- Sedentary women: 1600 daily calories
- Moderately active women: 1800 daily calories
- Active women: 2000 to 2200 daily calories

These guidelines are for 50+ women who would like to maintain a healthy weight and remain fit. Knowing your daily calorie needs gives insight into the number of hours you can put into fasting weekly while giving your body what it needs. If you are active or moderately active and you plan to lose weight healthily, aim to consume about 1200 calories daily. This will help you lose up to 2 pounds per week.

Get Familiar with Your Numbers

Before you start any weight loss plan, calculate your body mass index (BMI) and use the scale at home to weigh yourself. Don't stop at that, though. Some other numbers affect your looks as you get older.

The first is your waist circumference. In some women, hormonal changes do not cause weight gain. Instead, they change the way they carry weight on their body. So, even when you aren't gaining weight, you may look like you are. Your waistline could become bigger, giving the appearance of weight gain. Most women notice weight gain in their mid-sections.

The second number to be familiar with is your body fat percentage. The older you get, the more likely it is that your body composition will change. A dip in your testosterone levels causes the loss of muscle mass, which changes body composition. So, even if your weight remains the same, you might look fatty due to muscle loss.

Evaluate Your Lifestyle

As you get older and closer to retirement, your interests naturally shift toward more leisurely activities. You may spend more time indulging yourself by entertaining friends, eating out in restaurants, reading, and generally practicing self-care. This is normal and understandable, but several of these activities may lead to weight gain if you aren't cautious.

To lose weight healthily, don't give up activities you enjoy, but making small changes and adjustments to your lifestyle can make all the difference. It can help alter your energy balance. For instance, if you like traveling, consider going on an active vacation rather than choosing a food-based cruise. If you enjoy cooking, spend your time in a healthy cooking class.

Eating in restaurants, entertaining friends, and increased travel could also mean you consume alcoholic beverages more frequently. Alcoholic calories add up more quickly than food calories, and they often add up in the mid-section. Additionally, it is difficult to make healthy food choices when you drink.

The bottom line is that you may need to eliminate alcohol from your diet or at least cut back on drinking if you want to reach your weight loss goals.

Get 8-Hours of Sleep Daily

Getting enough sleep is essential for people of all ages, but particularly for women over 50. Sleep helps regulate the hormones in charge of your appetite. It also enhances brain and cognitive function, prevents injury, and energizes you to stay active throughout the day.

Obese and overweight people get less sleep than those who do not fall into that category. When you regularly deprive yourself of sleep, your body automatically increases hormones such as cortisol and ghrelin. Respectively, these hormones increase hunger and stimulate the appetite.

Older women who get less than five hours of sleep every night are twice as likely to be overweight or obese as those who get a solid 7 to 8 hours of sleep a night. Therefore, having a consistent sleep schedule isn't only an excellent idea. It is a necessity for anyone looking to lose weight. Being consistent means you wake up and retire to bed around the same time every day. If you don't make this a habit, you stand the risk of becoming obese.

The CDC recommends 7 to 9 hours of sleep a night for women in their fifties.

Know Your Macronutrients

Three primary macronutrients are essential for healthy and effective weight loss after age 50. They are Carbohydrates, Protein, and Dietary Fat. Carb and protein give the body four calories per gram, while dietary fat provides nine calories per gram.

Based on the Institute of Medicine recommendations, women over 50 should get 45 to 65 percent of their daily calories from carbs, 10 to 35 percent from protein, and 20 to 35 percent from dietary fat.

Since protein and dietary fiber are known to promote satiety, which is necessary for weight loss, consider the following when consuming your daily 1200 calories:

- 40% of calories from carbs, which is 120g of carbs daily.

- 35% of calories from protein, which equals 105g of protein daily

- 25% of calories from dietary fat, which is 40g of fat daily

If you don't have the time to count macronutrient grams, try dividing your plate during mealtime. Doing that will make sure that you get your daily nutritional needs. It is an excellent way to properly portion your meals and get all the essential nutrients to stay optimally healthy while you are on the path to losing the extra pounds.

Increase Daily Physical Activities

Exercise and workouts are not the only ways to get active every day. You can increase the number of calories your body burns daily by getting certain activities done. This is a surefire way to promote weight loss or maintenance after age 50.

The following are a few activities and how many calories you'll burn in 30 minutes:

- Dancing: 112 calories
- Cooking: 93 calories
- Bowling: 112 calories
- Gardening: 167 calories
- House cleaning: 167 calories
- Horseback riding: 149 calories
- Weeding: 172 calories
- Painting: 186 calories
- Raking: 149 calories

The point is to avoid sitting down as much as you can throughout the day. Since you now know how many calories each activity can help burn, calculate how many calories you want to burn and put in the work. Even if you have to get a sit/stand desk at work, increase your physical activities.

Drink Plenty of Non-Calorie Drinks

Drinking plenty of water every day will prevent dehydration and reduce hunger. In the morning, try to drink up to four cups of water when you wake up. Do that before you consume your morning tea or coffee. Also, drink 2 cups of water before breakfast as this helps to boost satiety.

Several studies have shown that caffeine aids fat-burning and weight loss. It also improves mental alertness and provides the boost of energy you need to stay active throughout each day. To reap its fat loss benefits, try to drink at least 3 cups of coffee or tea each day—no need to fret because 500 mg of caffeine every day is considered safe for the average adult.

Balance Your Daily Workouts

Any exercise on a day-to-day basis is an excellent idea for most people. But in your fifties, you need to take a more balanced approach to workouts. In fact, having a balanced exercise and workout program is one of the most important things. With a balanced program, you can offset most hormonal changes and body composition issues that arise with aging.

You can work out however you deem fit, but any program you follow should contain the four elements below:

- **Strength Training** – Resistance training exercises aim to enhance muscle growth and development. Doing them will keep your metabolism healthy. Multiple studies have confirmed that strength training has age-related benefits for older people.

- **Flexibility Training** – This involves stretching exercises targeted at increasing your joints' motion range. Daily flexibility training will help you stay limber and comfortable as you juggle through your daily living activities.

- **Aerobic Training** – Daily cardiovascular activities regulate the decrease in metabolic rate, which comes with age. More importantly, they also help to improve heart health. Combined with intermittent fasting, they can help to manage heart health risks.

- **Stability Training** – Including functional training activities in your daily routine will help you maintain a stable, healthy, and youthful body and look. Stability exercises are fortunately simple and take minutes to perform. Daily workouts can help improve your posture, balance, and overall appearance.

More workouts and exercises will be discussed later in the book. In the section about exercise for women over 50, you will determine your workout routine's specific activities.

The ideal approach is to make a total of three changes as you include everything discussed here in your daily routine. Adding over three can make you feel overwhelmed, and you might even be tempted to end your weight loss journey.

Remember that everyone ages differently, so don't compare yourself to anyone else in your age group. Be kind to yourself as your body changes, but don't stop motivating yourself to stay smart and active and keep your body lean and healthy as you add more years to your age.

Mindful Eating

Mindfulness is a habit we must all cultivate. Mindful eating is one thing every dieter should have in their toolbox. Often, mindless eating results from stress. Improving your awareness of what you eat can help you manage your weight better.

Mindful eating is all about paying attention as you plan your meals and eat them. It helps you know how hungry or full you are to avoid overeating or under-eating. Using this technique means you leave your phone or newspaper when you eat. This fully immerses you in the present. By using the mindful eating technique, you can tell exactly how your foods taste. But the most important thing is that making mindful eating a way of life can make your weight loss goals more achievable.

The North Carolina State University conducted an online mindfulness-based weight-loss study which confirmed that individuals who practice mindfulness eating lost more weight on average than those in a standard food control group. This study was presented at the European Congress on Obesity.

Foods That Promote Healthy Weight Loss in Women Over 50

As crucial as mindful eating is to healthy weight loss, eating the right food is also essential. What you eat is just as important as when you eat and what you do when eating. As you grow older, your body requires more specific foods and vitamins. It is usual for nutritional needs to change over different phases in life.

In youth, your nutritional requirements are geared toward growth and maintaining your body for procreation, should that be a goal for you. After age 50, they become targeted at keeping your mind and body in an optimal state of health. This, of course, includes leaving the extra fat off and looking as fit as possible.

Maintaining optimal health depends on what you eat. As you age, what you eat becomes more important than ever. Remember that your metabolic rate drops when you reach the 50-years mark. You need to consume foods that your body will find easier to break down and convert to fuel instead of adding them to the fat storage.

And some vitamins become more vital to protect you against diseases and general or specific health issues. Thus, you are responsible for making sure the foods you consume the most contain those essential vitamins that your body requires to stay healthy.

Shown below are foods that should be a part of your diet to keep your mind sharp and your body strong as you get rid of unwanted fat storage.

• Fiber-Rich Foods

You have likely learned the importance of fiber-rich foods from experience, as most people do. Gastrointestinal function declines in older people. Due to this, you must focus on consuming sufficient fiber to keep the system running smoothly.

Not only does fiber aid gastrointestinal function operate without hiccups, but it also reduces inflammation and cholesterol. It does all this while ensuring a release of energy-filled carbs into your bloodstream.

Ensure that you eat as much as 30g of fiber daily to keep your system going at a healthy pace. Raspberries, lentils, whole-wheat pasta, and green peas are a few of the richest fiber sources.

• B12 Foods

Stomach acidity decreases as the body ages. Getting enough B12 vitamins in your diet becomes harder. Stomach acid aids the release of B12 from the foods you eat to maintain your nervous system's health. This also helps critical metabolic processes.

Over the age of 50, approximately 10-30% of women experience difficulty absorbing the B12 from their foods. Those who are on medications that suppress stomach acid especially find it harder to get B12 from goods. On average, you should get up to 2.4 micrograms of this essential vitamin per day.

Dairy and foods from animals, such as meat, seafood, and egg, contain high amounts of vitamin B12. But you can also get it from your whole-grain cereals and other B12-fortified foods. If you have reason to believe that you are not getting adequate B12, discuss your concerns with your doctor, and they will probably recommend a B12 supplement or multivitamin to include in your diet.

- **Potassium-Rich Foods**

Bananas are probably the most popular source of potassium. It is commonly known that the risk of heart disease and stroke increases with age. An excellent way to lower the risk is to consume foods that are excellent sources of potassium. Examples include bananas and avocados.

The World Health Organization suggests that potassium can play a pivotal role in lowering the risks associated with blood pressure. The recommendation from the WHO says that women over 50 should consume a daily 4700 mg of potassium.

Besides bananas or avocados, potatoes and pistachios are also good sources of potassium. One potato contains around 900 mg of potassium. A cup of pistachios contains 1200 mg, an avocado has over 700 mg per cup, and a single banana has 400 mg.

- **Calcium-Rich Foods**

Calcium is recognized as the number one go-to nutrient for anyone looking to build and maintain strong bones and teeth. But most people don't know that it is key to the heart's function. Not only that, but it also helps make sure that the muscles and nervous system function as efficiently as they should.

The goal is for any woman over 50 to consume at least 1200 mg of calcium every day. But intake may sometimes be an issue due to two things. The first is that lactose-intolerant people may have a problem getting enough calcium, especially as they age. The second thing is that insufficient vitamin D in the body makes it hard to absorb calcium. Note that vitamin D also helps to boost immune function.

Scientific research has shown that as a person ages, access to vitamin D through sunlight and other fatty foods, added to the inability to absorb vitamins as efficiently as before, results in significantly below-standard levels of this essential vitamin.

The key to combatting these two problems is to consume more leafy greens such as kale, mustard, collards, and bok choy. You may also add sardines and canned salmon and tofu made with a calcium compound to your diet.

You may also need to ask your doctor to check your vitamin D level to know if you are getting enough vitamins. The consensus is that women should be within 70 nmol/L. If you don't have enough vitamin D, try getting at least 15 minutes of sunlight every day. Also, take any supplement recommendations from your doctor.

- **Turmeric and Cinnamon**

One other thing changes as you get older – taste. With age comes a decline in the production of saliva and your ability to perceive taste. To avoid losing that ability completely, consider experimenting with spices such as turmeric.

Research has shown that turmeric boosts immune function and reduces inflammation in the joints, preventing arthritis in older women. The main compound in turmeric is curcumin, which scientific studies suggest may have an authentic effect on certain forms of cancer and even Alzheimer's.

Cinnamon is another spice that should go into your cooking rotation. It is recognized as a potent anti-inflammatory and anti-microbial agent. It also helps regulate blood sugar levels by slowing the rate at which the tummy empties after meals. You may also use cinnamon therapeutically to manage your body's sensitivity to type 2 diabetes.

Besides making these important foods a part of your cooking plan for your eating windows, also follow these general guidelines for healthy eating. Sticking to them will help in your quest to lose weight healthily.

- Reduce saturated fats from your diet. Doing that will decrease the risk of cardiovascular disease. Eat more healthy fats derived from lean meats, low-fat dairy, fish, olive oil, nuts, and plant-based foods like avocado.

- Minimize or eliminate processed foods and drinks from your diet. Some of these include cookies, candies, chips, cakes, and pastries. Refined foods are known to increase inflammation in the body, leading to an increased risk of diabetes, cancer, and heart disease.

Follow every tip discussed. You can fast, lose weight, and stay fit, all while maintaining desirable physical and mental health.

Chapter 6: Hormones and Weight Loss

Hormones are chemicals secreted in the endocrine system by the glands. They travel through the bloodstream to your tissue and organs, telling them what to do and when to do it. They are crucial to regulating most of the primary bodily functions and processes, and they have an undeniable impact on your overall functioning.

Hormones do their jobs well when they are in a balanced state. But sometimes, they can become too much or too little in the bloodstream. This is when hormonal imbalance occurs. Due to the vital role hormones play in the body, a slight imbalance in hormonal secretion can trigger a ripple effect throughout your body.

Hormonal imbalance is one of the leading causes of weight gain in women over age 50. Add it to other factors that come with menopause, and weight loss becomes an almost unachievable goal for older women. Unexplained weight gain or weight loss (depending on whether the hormone is oversecreted or under-secreted) is the leading sign of imbalanced hormones.

Everyone experiences naturally driven periods of imbalance in hormone production. Fluctuations typically occur at different points in life. Sometimes, improper functioning of the endocrine system causes imbalance.

There are different endocrinal glands across the body, and they are all responsible for other organs. Some include:

- Adrenal glands
- Hypothalamus glands
- Thyroid and parathyroid glands
- Pituitary glands
- Pineal gland
- Gonads
- Pancreatic islets

Varying medical conditions can affect some of these endocrinal glands. Lifestyle habits and certain environmental factors may also play a role in hormonal imbalance, but sometimes, it just happens with age.

Many changes you experience between 40 and 50, such as menopause and decreased metabolism, are caused by a decline in hormone production. This naturally happens with age and has a significant impact on weight gain or loss. Increased hunger due to the overdrive in appetite hormones is a common symptom of a hormonal condition.

Sometimes, weight gain in your older age has nothing to do with eating habits or exercise routines. For most women over 50, misfiring hormones are the leading reason behind the unwanted pounds adding up.

To lose weight, you have to harmonize your hormone levels, and this requires focusing on more than one hormone. Interestingly, many people assume that estrogen is the only hormone that matters when managing weight issues in menopausal age, but it is far from the fact.

But first, how can you be sure that your hormones are responsible for the new extra weight? There are signs to watch out for. Getting familiar with these signs can help you identify the exact cause of weight gain so you can work on a targeted solution.

- **Bigger Waistline While Eating Right**

Suppose love handles suddenly appear around your waist even though you've had a reasonably flat tummy for the majority of your life. This is the number one sign that hormonal imbalance is at work. As you age, your body becomes more resistant to insulin. That drives it to store instead of burning fat.

Also, your estrogen becomes more dominant as you enter your perimenopause stage and beyond, leading to even more insulin resistance. All these cause your belly fat to build up and your waist to become bigger.

- **Your Sugar Craving Increases**

Insulin resistance can increase diabetes risk, but that is not all it does. It also affects other vital hormones. For instance, insulin resistance affects leptin, the hormone that lets your body know when your stomach is full—the higher your insulin resistance, the more your leptin levels increase.

Increased leptin, regardless of what you think, does not make you put down the spoon and stop eating. Instead, it results in dysfunctional leptin receptors. When not functioning correctly, the receptors stop alerting your brain when you are full. Due to that, you do the direct opposite of what your leptin is designed to regulate. In other words, you continue eating because your brain does not send the signal to stop.

• Frequent Mood Swings

As you reach the perimenopausal age and eventually the post-menopausal age, estrogen levels start fluctuating frequently. The results of this are mood swings and weight gain in your belly. It explains why women are more susceptible to mood disorders than men.

A study conducted by the University of Wisconsin on the Neurobiological Underpinnings of the Estrogen found that women's estrogen levels fluctuate more frequently during menopausal transitions and reproductive cycle events. This also tends to be the time when women report depression and recurrent depression the most.

Estrogen levels naturally fluctuate during menopause, leading to mood swings and weight gain. More light will be shed on this later in this chapter.

• Never-Ending Stress

If you find you are always stressed, that means your cortisol hormone is on overdrive. As you might know, cortisol is also called the stress hormone. It often increases when your body senses overwhelming anxiety and may cause stubborn weight gain, particularly in your midsection.

When you experience high levels of stress and anxiety, your body triggers the fight-or-flight response, which you may call the "survival mode." Cortisol production increases when this happens, and your body receives signals to do more storing and less burning of fat.

• Exhaustion Without Sleep

Exhaustion and insomnia are possible signs that hormones are responsible for your weight gain. So, look out for them. Not getting adequate sleep can cause fatigue, which results in stress-induced insomnia. All of these affect your hormone production, especially cortisol levels.

Increased cortisol production causes thyroid production to decrease, which leads to central weight gain. It can also affect the hormones in charge of muscle growth, tissue building, and overall health.

To help you better understand how much effect your hormones can have on weight gain and weight loss, more specific insight will be provided on each hormone mentioned so far and others and how they influence fat storage in the body.

At least five hormones experience imbalance and affect your ability to metabolize appropriately once you reach menopause. Together, they sabotage your weight loss efforts and make you believe that you can no longer get rid of extra fats. These five hormones are:

- Estrogen
- Cortisol
- Thyroid
- Testosterone
- Insulin

One by one, let's delve deeper into these hormones and how they can influence your weight loss journey as a woman trying to burn fat and stay fit in your fifties.

Estrogen

When you hear the word "estrogen," you probably think of a single hormone. Contrary to most people's beliefs, estrogen consists of three major hormones – estriol, estradiol, and estrone.

Estrogen is one of the primary sex hormones in females, but men also secrete it, although in smaller amounts. Declining estrogen levels affect men's waistlines just as they affect women's waistlines in later years.

Women naturally produce higher amounts of estrogen, which shapes their unique hourglass figure. But with age, estrogen levels decrease, causing women to assume a more masculine shape and figure.

Estrogen is also one hormone that causes women challenges in the fat department as they get older. Out-of-balance estrogen levels can turn the average woman into a fat-storing machine. This sometimes happens rapidly, leaving a woman feeling frustrated and confused.

Estrogen does not work alone. It operates in tandem with a group of steroid hormones known as progesterone. Your progesterone levels also decline with age. The symptoms typically include breast swelling, mood swings, trouble sleeping, irritability, and water retention.

If you have the coveted hourglass shape, that is courtesy of estrogen. This hormone is in charge of storing and regulating fat in the hips and thighs. When working together, progesterone and estrogen stop the body from storing fat around the waist, providing that tiny waist women like to flaunt. Still, the harmonious relationship between both sometimes suffers interference.

Stress affects the progesterone's function, leading to weight gain in and around the belly. The fat here is usually difficult to shift because progesterone levels are lower than estrogen levels in most women.

High levels of stress and anxiety negatively impact the production of progesterone. So, when you notice fat accumulating around your waist area without you increasing your calorie intake or reducing physical activity, that is a sign you need to cut down on the stress-inducing events in your day-to-day life. Doing that will help keep progesterone levels balanced.

Since estrogen production decline rarely happens until later in life, women believe that excess estrogen is a good thing. Unfortunately, that is not the case. Estrogen dominance can lead to excessive weight gain when progesterone isn't at the same levels.

When your body produces too much estrogen, you cannot reap the positive effects of progesterone. This is because the overproduction of estrogen leads to overstimulation of the brain and body.

The confusion around estrogen-progesterone partnership arises when you find that your estrogen levels are low, but you are estrogen-dominant anyway. Dominance occurs when an estrogen to progesterone ratio is higher than usual. That means you need more progesterone to keep estrogen levels from acting erratically.

How do you know when you are estrogen-dominant in your fifties?

- Weight gain in the abdomen and hips area
- Inability to lose weight easily
- Bloating
- Water retention
- Mood swings
- Slow metabolism
- Fatigue
- Trouble sleeping

If you notice that your weight gain isn't responding to dietary changes or workout routines, below is a quick quiz you can take to check if estrogen is dominating progesterone in an imbalanced way.

Do you sweat a lot at night?

o Yes, every night

o Once a week

o 3 to 5 times a week

o Never

Do you have hot flushes?

    o Once a day

    o 5 times a day or more

    o 1 to 5 times a day

o Never

Have you gained a lot of weight recently?

    o Yes

    o No

Do you experience abnormal periods?

    o Yes

    o No

o Used to experience abnormal periods but no longer have periods

Do you suffer from low libido?

    o Yes

    o No

Do you experience bloating?

    o Yes

    o No

o Occasionally

Do you have food cravings?

    o Yes

    o No

    o Sometimes

Your answers to these questions will help you determine whether you have estrogen dominance based on what you have learned about its symptoms. Eventually, you will discover how intermittent fasting can help you manage hormonal imbalances to promote healthy weight loss. But meanwhile, let's move on to the next hormone that affects weight gain and loss.

Cortisol

So far, you know how cortisol affects weight loss, but let's go deeper to explore the relationship between both. Earlier, you learned that cortisol is the body's stress hormone. Its production increases when the body activates the survival mode, otherwise known as the fight or flight response.

Elevated stress causes an imbalance in your cortisol, adrenaline, and DHEA hormones. High-stress levels stimulate your adrenal glands, helping to excessively produce all these hormones. When the stress levels drop, hormones should naturally balance out. However, occasionally, the hormones remain irregular for prolonged periods, causing a ripple of adverse effects on your body. That, unfortunately, includes weight gain.

Of all these hormones, cortisol has the strongest link with weight fluctuation in older women. Excess or deficiency of the hormone can affect your thyroid functions and blood sugar levels, which triggers signs of slow metabolism and weight fluctuation.

The major stressors that may contribute to cortisol imbalance are:

- Inadequate sleep
- Emotional imbalances
- Excessive carb intake
- Inconsistent work schedule
- Frequent delay of meals
- Toxin exposure

Cortisol has an exciting and vital relationship with insulin, which controls your blood sugar levels. An increase in cortisol levels promotes insulin resistance, which causes blood sugar levels to suffer instability. This typically leads to weight gain, higher blood sugar and increases the risk of type 2 diabetes.

On the other hand, cortisol levels can also dramatically decrease. This is known as adrenal exhaustion. When it happens, blood sugar levels decline, resulting in hypoglycemia. This condition is linked to unhealthy weight loss and decreased stress tolerance.

Increased or decreased imbalance in cortisol levels can cause metabolism to decline, particularly in women over 50. To a significant extent, cortisol levels are also responsible for the optimal production of hormones in the thyroid gland.

When the thyroid gland functions correctly, it helps to maintain a healthy metabolism, regardless of age. But imbalanced cortisol levels can potentially impair the body's ability to convert inactive thyroid to its active form. Again, this can lead to a decreased thyroid problem, leading to low metabolism and unwanted weight gain.

To address the hormonal imbalance that concerns your cortisol and thyroid, you may need to consult your doctor, who will advise you on the best steps to identify the exact issue responsible for low metabolism and weight gain.

After this, you can work with your doctor to discuss diet recommendations, which could be intermittent fasting, plus other lifestyle changes and the introduction of nutritional supplements to your daily routine.

Thyroid

The thyroid gland is one of the glands in your endocrine system. Its job is to produce the thyroid hormones, which go into your bloodstream and transmit to your tissues and organs to help your body put energy to use. The point of this is to help the brain, heart, muscles, and several other organs function as efficiently as they should keep your body running without hitches. So, thyroid hormones are quite important. Now, what is the nature of the relationship between thyroid hormones and weight?

Medical experts have affirmed an intricate relationship between thyroid disease, metabolism, and body weight for a long time. Thyroid hormones regulate metabolism. You can determine your metabolism by measuring the amount of oxygen your body uses over a specific timeframe.

This measurement, if made at rest, is called the basal metabolic rate (BMR). The BMR is one of the earliest ways of assessing thyroid status in patients. Those with nonfunctioning thyroid glands were discovered to have low BMRs, and those with overactive thyroid glands had higher BMRs.

Later, advanced research linked the initial observations with the measurements of thyroid hormone levels. They found that low thyroid levels were associated with low BMRs, and high thyroid levels were connected with high BMRs. The BMR measurement isn't used as much nowadays due to the test's complexity. Still, it does establish a link between weight and thyroid state.

People with hyperthyroidism, which is when the thyroid glands are overactive, have elevated BMRs. Those with overactive thyroid hormones experience weight loss, which can be extreme in some cases. Furthermore, weight loss is influenced by the extent of the thyroid's overactivity.

This means that when the thyroid becomes hyperactive, the BMR increases, meaning that a person has to consume more calories to maintain their body weight. If the number of calories isn't increased to match the excess calories burned, it will cause extreme weight loss.

As indicated before, the factors that regulate appetite, activity, and metabolism are complex. At the center of this complex system is the thyroid hormone. But on average, the more severe hyperthyroidism is, the more extreme the weight loss is.

Hyperthyroidism is an abnormal state, which is why it promotes unhealthy weight loss. Suppose you are losing weight in your 50s, even without dieting or anything. There, the right thing to do is to check for any possible imbalance in your thyroid hormones.

Naturally, any weight loss caused by an overactive thyroid will eventually go away when you treat and reverse the condition. However, this is tricky. If you continue eating more calories, it can cause excess weight gain.

On the other hand, hypothyroidism – which refers to underactive thyroid gland activity, has a relationship with weight gain. BMR is typically lower in people with underactive thyroid hormones, which lead to weight gain.

The amount of weight gained often depends on the severity of hypothyroidism. But the decline in BMR due to underactive thyroid is much less extreme than the increase experienced in hyperthyroidism. This leads to more slight alterations in weight.

The exact cause of weight gain in hypothyroid people is tricky. It sometimes has nothing to do with calorie or fat accumulation. Most times, the excess weight happens due to the accumulation of water and salt. Rarely does massive weight gain happen due to hypothyroidism.

Generally, most people don't gain more than ten pounds of fat due to the thyroid, depending on the gland's level of inactivity. If weight gain is the only present sign of hypothyroidism, your weight gain likely has little to do with the thyroid.

Thyroid hormones have been used as a tool for healthy weight loss. Increasing thyroid hormone to elevate the hormone levels may not cause a dramatic weight change. But thyroid hormone treatment can help achieve more weight loss than some dieting plans. Naturally, you have to talk with your doctor to determine if you need the treatment. However, fasting can help you achieve balance in production to avoid gaining unwanted excess weight.

Testosterone

Testosterone may be the primary sex hormone in men, but it is present abundantly in women too. It may not be as much, but it certainly plays some vital role, particularly for losing fat.

This hormone is responsible for muscle growth in both men and women. Testosterone deficiency automatically makes you predisposed to excessive fat storage. To understand and manage testosterone imbalance, it's essential to understand its role in weight gain and fat loss.

One crucial function of this hormone is to build and maintain muscle mass and promote muscle growth. It also boosts bone strength. Your hormonal levels decline as you add years, which is why muscle and bone loss occurs the older you get.

Just as it promotes muscle growth, testosterone also suppresses fat gain. So, when the levels decline, its fat-suppressing ability declines as well. As a result, you may start gaining more fat than you want.

As explained earlier, muscles use way more calories than fat tissue. With the loss of muscle in older women, you are at the risk of overeating and storing extra calories as body fat. This means that reduced muscle mass due to testosterone decline or deficiency is the primary reason older women start gaining extra pounds with age.

Here's where it gets interesting – obesity may suppress testosterone levels in older women. Multiple studies have shown that obese women have lower testosterone levels than normal-weight ones. Therefore, excessive fat storage in the body may suppress your testosterone levels.

The key to preventing weight gain due to low testosterone levels is to work on increasing them naturally. The number one sign of decline in older women is reduced muscle mass. So, if you lose muscles at an alarming rate, your testosterone might be dangerously low. There, there are natural steps you can take to drive the levels up to aid weight loss.

A few include:

- Getting enough vitamin D
- Eating zinc-rich foods
- Getting adequate sleep
- Minimizing the stressors in your daily life and environment
- Strength training

When you combine these with intermittent fasting and other effective weight loss techniques, these steps will get your testosterone levels back up so you can lose weight without worries.

The right thing to do if you suspect you have testosterone deficiency is to reach out to your doctor. A simple blood test will reveal the truth, and your doctor will tell you the next step. He or she may recommend testosterone replacement therapy, which is frankly the best way to stabilize your hormonal levels. But this should only be a resort if the natural methods do not work for you.

Insulin

Insulin and weight gain usually go hand in hand. The more insulin your body produces, the more likely you are to add extra pounds. Still, weight control or loss is not entirely impossible. You have only to normalize your insulin levels to reduce or avoid weight gain.

Insulin is much misunderstood. Too little insulin in the bloodstream can cause serious health problems, and too much can cause weight gain. A general side effect for those who take insulin is weight gain.

Therefore, if you have any condition that requires you to take insulin, you are more prone to weight gain. Add that to age-triggered weight gain, and you realize that you have a lot to do if you want to lose weight effectively.

How does insulin contribute to weight gain?

When you take insulin, glucose enters your cells, making your blood glucose levels drop. That is how insulin treatment is supposed to work. But consider you consume more calories than you need to achieve a healthy weight, depending on your activity level. In that case, your cells might end up getting more glucose than necessary. This means that they can't use it all. Glucose not used by the cells eventually stores as fat in the body.

Note that insulin does not precisely stop your body from burning fat. But it does have a significant influence on the rate at which fat burns. That is because, apart from insulin being the body's blood glucose regulator, it also:

- **Inhibits Lipolysis**

Throughout lipolysis, accumulated fatty acids move out of your fat cells into the bloodstream, where they are used for energy. When insulin levels are high, it inhibits this process by blocking the release of fatty acids, thus ensuring that you get fewer fatty acids to fuel your metabolically active tissues. Due to this, your body's ability to burn fat is significantly reduced.

- **Initiates Lipogenesis**

Lipogenesis is when fatty acids move from your bloodstream into your fat cells, where they are stored away for later use. Many people call this the "fat storage mode," and they try as much as possible to avoid it.

Besides, lipogenesis can cause carbohydrates to convert and store as fat. This process is called Novo lipogenesis. Novo lipogenesis only happens when there is a surplus of carbs and calories, usually in meaningful amounts. You consistently burn fewer calories than you eat. As a result, insulin can sometimes be a strong villain in your quest to burn and lose fat.

The key is to keep your insulin as low as possible to lose weight healthily. Without doing that, you might keep adding extra pounds. Eating fewer calories can help you keep your insulin levels down. That is why intermittent fasting is such an ideal dieting strategy for weight loss.

If done the right way, intermittent fasting can help you manage most hormonal imbalances responsible for weight gain in your older age. It increases insulin resistance. Doing that helps your cells recognize insulin more effectively, tapping into the fat-burning mechanism that allows natural weight loss.

Fasting increases the growth hormone, one of the crucial hormones your body needs to burn fat and increase muscle mass. You can't immediately detect your growth hormone levels when you eat. If you always eat and snack from daybreak until you retire to bed, you aren't giving your growth hormone the breather it needs to repair your muscle mass. On the other hand, Fasting can help minimize the rate at which you eat, causing your hormone to increase by up to 2000 percent.

Finally, intermittent fasting decreases cortisol levels and increases melatonin. Cortisol is the stress hormone, while melatonin is the sleep hormone. A balance in your cortisol and melatonin levels can be achieved with intermittent fasting and a proper workout routine. You need balanced melatonin to sleep and rest. When your melatonin levels are stabilized, you don't have to worry about insomnia and not getting enough sleep.

High levels of the sleep hormone make you feel dizzy and tired, so you can rest until the morning. Then, cortisol gives the mental awareness and energy you require to get the day going after you wake.

And when you are well-rested, other hormones responsible for weight loss and weight gain are positively affected. So, using intermittent fasting to balance your cortisol and melatonin is a win-win situation.

Homeostasis is vital for good health and wellness. It is your key to feeling and looking good. Paired with proper nutrients and a healthy workout program, intermittent fasting can help you achieve homeostasis to promote weight loss even as you get older.

Intermittent fasting is just one way of balancing your hormones. Besides this, there are other things you can do. You can redefine your diet and make sure it is filled with food that regulates and balances your hormone levels.

- **Carbs:** Don't stop eating carbs because you believe they contribute to weight gain. Well, you may stop eating carbs, but only the bad ones. Add more "good" carbs to your diet. Examples of good carbs include unprocessed whole grains, beans, vegetables, and fruit.

- **Organic:** Be more organic with your food choices to keep your hormones balanced. Organic foods and drinks are typically devoid of growth hormones. Also, it is believed that pesticides contribute to hormonal disruption in older and younger women. Add more root vegetables and leafy greens to your diet as they give your body the complex carbs it needs.

- **Kale:** Eating kale is excellent, but too much of it can disrupt your hormones. It is best to consume cruciferous vegetables as moderately as you can. Kale contains goitrogens, which can block iodine from entering your thyroid gland.

Your body requires iodine to secret the thyroid hormones, which are necessary for normal metabolism. More dairy in your diet can help you get enough iodine into your thyroid gland. But this doesn't mean you should skip out on kale totally. You can still eat it, but don't make it too much.

- **Probiotics and Prebiotics:** Gut health is crucial to hormonal balance. Unbalanced hormones affect your microbiome and gut barrier. This can cause inflammation issues. Add more probiotics food like yogurt, sauerkraut, and fermented foods to your diet. Also, prebiotics such as asparagus, bananas, and shiitake mushrooms should be a constant. All of these will keep your hormones balanced and your guts healthy.

- **Healthy Fats:** The AARP recommends that consuming more healthy fats such as olive oil, coconut oil, avocados, and sweet potatoes can help maintain estrogen levels balanced in the body. So, add more of these to your diet as well.

To wrap it up, ensure you eat less sugar, gluten, dairy, etc. You don't have to get rid of them. Just limit your consumption of them, as overeating can spike your insulin levels and disrupt other hormones crucial to keeping fit.

Hormones have a massive impact on the body's functioning. However, they decline with age, then affecting what they impact. To keep your body and mind healthy and sound, your hormones have to be balanced.

Imbalance in hormones can lead to many issues, including weight gain. That is precisely why you should be familiar with them and learn how you can manage hormonal imbalance to achieve your weight loss goals, regardless of aging.

Chapter 7: The First Days of Intermittent Fasting

Getting started with intermittent fasting can be arduous if you have never gone hungry for a prolonged period. The very idea is daunting. It's normal for people to think, "Oh, I can't do this. I won't last the day. I give up" before fasting at all. But these negative thoughts will be much less prominent in your head when you know what to expect.

What are the first few days of intermittent fasting like? How long does it take your body to acclimatize with the new routine? What are the side-effects you might experience when you start fasting? The answers to these and many other questions will give you an insight into what to expect as you begin periodic fasting.

First, do not see intermittent fasting as a duty or task you owe your health and body. That just takes the fun out of everything. Instead, consider it a self-experiment – something you are doing to get to know more about your body and what makes it tick.

Break down your plan into small, doable actions that can be achieved step-by-step. That way, you can be guaranteed to finish with the program. As the fasting days go by, ensure you observe, analyze, and put down what you discover about your body and intermittent fasting. At the end of the fasting period, make your conclusion as to whether intermittent fasting is right for you.

Doing it that way makes it less of something to commit to and more of something to learn about. So, it doesn't feel like a task you have to endure. Instead, it feels like a process you are gaining knowledge from. This method makes it easy for you to start and finish your intermittent fasting plan. As humans, we learn best by doing.

There are different fasting stages, and they all have various hallmark features, as you will notice when you begin. What does each entail?

Fed State

The fed state is the first stage of fasting, and it is initiated within the early few hours after your eating window. It occurs as your body digests and breaks down nutrients from food for absorption. During this stage, your blood sugar levels rise, and your body secretes high amounts of insulin.

The insulin level in your bloodstream depends on your meal's composition, the number of carbs you ate, and your body's sensitivity to insulin. Extra glucose is stored in muscles and the liver as glycogen. Meanwhile, the levels of leptin and ghrelin also change. Ghrelin levels decrease because you have just eaten. Remember that ghrelin stimulates hunger. Leptin, on the other hand, increases to suppress your appetite.

Remember that the stages in IF occur in a cycle. The fed-fast state resets back to the fed state if you consume food during the fasting window. This makes it impossible for your body to complete the whole cycle. Also, the provided state's duration depends on the composition and size of the meal you consumed.

Early Fasting State

Three to four hours after you eat, your body shifts into the early fasting state. This stage lasts until about 18 hours. In this phase, your insulin and blood sugar levels begin to decrease, pushing your body to start converting stored carbs (glycogen) into sugar to use as fuel.

As this phase nears its end, you will eventually run out of glycogen stores, and your body will start the search for another energy source. This heightens lipolysis, which is a process in which your body breaks down fat cells into smaller molecules so they can serve as an alternative energy source. At the same time, your body converts amino acids into energy.

Most of the intermittent fasting plans explained in chapter three-cycle are between the first stage (fed state) and the second stage (early fasting state).

Fasting State

To enter the fasting state, you must have fasted from around 18 hours to 2 days. So, if you fast today and skip fasting the next day, your body might not trigger the fasting state. By this stage, your body has completely depleted the glycogen stores and has broken down fat stores and protein for fuel.

The result is that your body produces ketone bodies – compounds produced when fat is converted into fuel. Your body goes into ketosis, which is a metabolic state where your body turns to fat as its primary energy source. But you might not transit into ketosis when you enter the fasting state. It sometimes happens later on.

As with the early fasting state, your last meal's size and composition determine how quickly your body transitions into ketosis. Individual differences may also play a part.

Common signs of ketosis include:

- Fatigue

- Fruity smelling breath

- Decreased appetite

- Weight loss

- A higher number of ketone bodies in your breath, blood, or urine,

Ketosis is the main result those who follow the ketogenic diet aim to achieve. By getting the body to reach ketosis, weight loss is achieved.

Note that shorter forms of intermittent fasting may not reach ketosis unless you follow a low-carb diet. By decreasing your carb intake, your body can quickly run out of glycogen and use fat as its primary fuel source.

Starvation State

You may also call this the long-term fasting state. After extended fasting periods, your body initiates this phase. It typically occurs around 48 hours after eating. In this state, insulin and blood sugar levels continue to drop, and beta-hydroxybutyrate (BHB) levels steadily rise. BHB is a type of ketone body.

In this same phase, your kidneys activate gluconeogenesis and generate sugar via this process. This serves as the primary fuel source for the brain. Ketone bodies also provide energy for your brain. The processing of branched-chain amino acids (BCAAS), some of the essential amino acids, is steadily reduced to conserve muscle tissue in the body. Understand that you shouldn't do long-term fasts unless your medical doctor gives the go-ahead.

These are the four phases you go through during intermittent fasting. Depending on the number of hours you fast, you may not reach some of these states in the fed-fast cycle.

Each phase changes the primary energy source for your body and hormones that concern metabolism.

How to Practice Fasting Safely

Unless you do it properly, fasting can pose a danger to your health. That is why you should know the right tips to follow when you start your fasting journey. Below are safety tips to ensure that your experience with intermittent fasting is smooth and seamless.

1. Make Fasting Periods Short

The duration of your fast is solely up to you. There are several techniques to choose from, so just select one that aligns with your lifestyle and daily living. Most regimens you have learned advise 8 to 24 hours of fasting. However, you can fast up to 72 hours if your doctor signals it is safe.

Remember that the longer your fasting window, the higher the risk of the side effects of fasting. Some of these include irritability, dehydration, hunger, fatigue, mood changes, fainting, and inability to focus.

The best thing is to stick to shorter fasting windows to avoid the side effects. This is especially important for you as a beginner and an older person. If you are confident in increasing your fasting time, ensure you seek your primary healthcare consultant's supervision.

• Eat Small Portions on Fast Days

Generally, the idea of fasting is to halt food and drink consumption for a specified period. When you start fasting, don't overcompensate for this by upping your regular food intake. Remember that intermittent fasting plans are based on calorie restriction. Therefore, eat as you usually do during your eating window.

Also, don't go for a full-blown fast where you eat nothing within your fast day. It is much safer to consume small amounts of food during fasting days. Taking this approach helps to lessen the risks associated with fasting. Fasting is also more sustainable since you are less likely to feel hungry.

- **Drink Water and Stay Hydrated**

Not drinking enough water can lead to dehydration, which can, in turn, lead to thirst, fatigue, and headaches. So, it is crucial to get enough fluid while fasting. Health authorities generally recommend following the 8x8 rule, so you drink 8-Ounces glasses of water every day. That is under 2 liters, and it will help you stay hydrated.

But know that the amount of fluid needed by the body can vary according to individuals. Still, most people's needs will likely fall in this range. Because up to 30 percent of required fluid comes from food, you can quickly become dehydrated while fasting.

On a fast, aim to drink two to three liters of water through the course of the day. Still, listen to your body to know when you are thirsty and need to drink more water.

- **Try Walking or Meditation**

It's challenging to avoid food during fasting windows, mainly if you are bored and hungry. If you don't play your cards right, you might break your fast unintentionally. One surefire way of preventing that is to keep yourself busy with brief walks or meditation.

These activities may help distract you from hunger without using too much of your energy. In general, any activity that is calming and mildly strenuous works because it will keep your mind engaged. You could read a book, listen to a podcast, or take a bath.

- **Don't Overeat When You Break Your Fast**

Unless you follow the warrior diet, you have no reason to consume a huge meal after the restriction is lifted. Even if you are on the warrior diet, you shouldn't necessarily "feast." Doing that can leave you feeling tired and bloated.

Also, feasting during eating windows can affect your long-term goals by inhibiting or slowing down your progress. As explained in an earlier chapter, your weight is affected by your total calorie quota. Thus, excessive calorie intake after a fast can decrease your calorie deficit.

Stick to your regular healthy eating routine even when you break a fast.

- **Stop Fasting if You Don't Feel Great**

It is normal to feel tired, irritable, and hunger during fasting windows – but feeling unwell isn't acceptable. If you are new to fasting, limit the restriction to below 24 hours. Keep a snack nearby if you feel faint or unwell.

If you become concerned about your health, stop fasting immediately. You might have to seek medical help if you experience severe tiredness or weakness to where you can't perform your daily tasks. Also, check for feelings of discomfort and sickness.

- **Don't Work Out Too Hard**

You might be able to maintain your standard exercise program while on a fast. That depends on you. But as a beginner to fasting, you are advised to keep exercise to the lowest intensity you can. Doing this will give insight into how much you can manage.

Low-intensity exercises such as mild yoga, walking, stretching, and housework are ideal for IF beginners. The most vital thing is to listen to your body. Rest if you experience any difficulty with exercise while on a fast. Keep your workout regimen as mild as needed.

Day 1-5 of Fasting

The steps below cover the first five days of fasting and what you should do during this period. This is specifically for the 16:8 plan, but you can tweak it to apply to the methods you want to follow.

Day 1: Don't Eat After Dinner

Eat as naturally as you do throughout the day but stop consuming anything once dinner is over. After dinner at 7 p.m., you are unlikely to be hungry around 8 to 9 p.m. But if you usually lounge around to watch TV or hang out with loved ones after dinner, you might nibble some popcorn, ice cream, or chips.

The tips below will help you through the night:

- Brush your teeth before bed. The minty taste from your toothpaste can help suppress cravings. Brushing also sends a subtle message to your brain you have finished eating, or you'll have to brush again. This creates enough of a barrier to keep you from eating.

- Drink a warm cup of herbal tea or a glass of water if you feel slightly hungry. The effect is calming.

- Go to bed and sleep the hunger off.

Day 2: Delay Breakfast

From the time you slept to the time you wake, you have effectively completed a 12-hour fast – but don't end it just yet. You have only balanced the ratio to 50:50, which is a good thing. That phase is straightforward, so you shouldn't feel it anyway.

It is morning, and there is the usual rush to get out of the house as soon as possible. Unless you work from home, the morning rush is a constant. You don't want to be late, so you grab something to eat on the go or eat as fast as possible. But when fasting, don't do this.

Delay your breakfast so you can eat when it is convenient, instead of rushing it. To make up for the delay, have a couple of glasses of water, coffee, or tea. You might think delaying breakfast is extreme or unhealthy, but it works.

Wait until you have settled in at work or dropped the kids off at school instead of eating amidst the early morning rush. Before you break your fast, check your mail, plan your day, and look at your calendar. Do not sneak in breakfast in the middle of these activities.

Once it is around 10 a.m., you can conveniently have your breakfast without all the chaos. Or, if you feel like you can manage, wait till 11 a.m. before you eat. But if you do eat around 10 a.m., you are unlikely to be hungry during lunchtime. Even though your clock says it's mealtime, your body might not agree. So, wait until you feel hungry again.

Around 2 p.m., you should be hungry; then you can have a nice lunch. Wait until 7 p.m. to have dinner. Then, repeat the steps above: don't eat after dinner and delay your breakfast until 10 a.m.

Day 3: Don't Snack

You have successfully completed a 15-hour fast. Your fasting window started after 7 p.m. the previous night. You ate nothing after dinner, and you delayed gratification (breakfast) until 10 a.m. That equals a whopping 15-hour fast, which is excellent for a beginner. After lunch on the third day, consume nothing until dinnertime. Leave snacks out of it.

- Dinner is just a few hours from lunch, so you can eat very soon. You only need to wait until 7 p.m.

- Hunger is temporary because it comes in waves. That means it will only subside the longer you go without food. It doesn't get worse.

- Sometimes, hunger is an illusion. It isn't real. You are not hungry – it might just be a snacking habit. Or maybe you are just hungry. You might be stressed, anxious, sad, bored, all of which can compel you to eat. Suppress the urge by drinking water, tea, or coffee instead.

- Keep yourself busy. Complete a task, go for a walk, meditate, or call a friend. Before you realize it, it will be time to head home and have your dinner.

Once you get home, cook your meal and eat at 7 p.m. Again, follow the previous steps: skip dinner, delay breakfast until 10 a.m., and don't snack until it's time for dinner.

Day 4: Skip Breakfast

By day 4, you have completed another 15-hour fast without snacking between meals. On the fourth day, skip breakfast by delaying mealtime for one more hour. This means having your first meal of the day at 11 a.m., making it lunch.

Repeat all the tips you have learned so far:

- Practice mindful eating by doing everything you need to do before your meal.

- Wait until you truly feel hungry before eating. Don't eat out of habit, thirst, or emotion.

- Understand that hunger is short-lived. Use tricks to ride hunger waves until they finally go away.

Again, have your dinner at 7 p.m. Repeat the steps you've followed from day 1 of fasting.

Day 5: Repeat

From day 1 to 4, you have built a routine that your body is starting to become familiar with. From day 5, just keep repeating the steps until you complete your plan. The 16:8 method reduces your eating window to one-third of the day, giving you a more generous fasting window to reap the benefits of intermittent fasting.

If you so wish, you can progress to other prolonged variations of intermittent fasting. Regardless of which techniques you choose to follow, always follow the principle of breaking down the fasting time into small, doable steps that can be easily achieved over some time. From there, work your way until you get to the exact point you want.

Fasting is an excellent tool for weight loss, but it can be even greater if you put yourself on a low-carb, high-fat diet while fasting. Its effectiveness depends on how consistent you are in the long run.

Should you follow the steps described in this section, it shouldn't be difficult to achieve consistency. One fun fact about skipping breakfast is that most people aren't starving in the morning, making it easy to skip breakfast without getting extremely hungry.

Chapter 8: Troubleshooting Intermittent Fasting

Varying factors contribute to how long it may take for you to start losing fat once you start intermittent fasting. Naturally, it varies from person to person, depending on starting weight, intermittent fasting approach taken, types and size of foods consumed during eating windows, and other factors.

Follow everything explained so far in this book by reducing your daily caloric intake and consistently expend more calories than you consume. Weight loss should start from the word "go." However, even though you are shedding the pounds, you may not notice the physical results for a couple of weeks. Most of the time, people just lose "water weight" in the beginner.

Depending on caloric intake during your fasting window, you may lose approximately 1 to 2 pounds each week. Hence, you would have to fast for up to 10 weeks to see any significant change in appearance.

If somehow, you are losing over two pounds per week, that could be a potential red flag. Contact your doctor immediately if you observe that you are losing a considerable amount of weight following a fasting plan. You might need to evaluate your daily or weekly caloric intake to establish that you are consuming enough nutrition to cater to your body's needs.

However, if you don't seem to be losing weight despite sticking to all the fasting guidelines, there could be different reasons. You could be making inevitable mistakes without realizing it. So, what could the mistakes be? Discover below.

High Caloric Intake During Eating Windows

The first likely reason could be that you are consuming too many calories during your eating window. As mentioned several times, weight loss via intermittent fasting boils down to the number of calories that go in versus the ones that come out. If you keep your caloric intake at the same number as before you started fasting, you can't possibly lose weight.

The whole point of intermittent fasting is restricting the time you eat to cut down on your calorie intake. Therefore, you can't keep packing in the same number of calories as before. If you do that, it means you haven't made any changes to your diet.

Solution: To fix this problem, get a calorie-counting app to track your intake for the first few days of intermittent fasting. With an app like that, you will know the exact number of calories you need to consume daily to lose weight. Usually, the estimations aren't wholly accurate, but they can make a difference initially. Some of these apps also have features that let you know the number of calories in most food. That way, you can plan your meal and adjust your diet.

Low Caloric Intake on Non-Fasting Days

Not consuming the required number of calories on non-fasting days makes your body conserve the consumed energy instead of burning it. Therefore, always endeavor to meet the daily caloric requirement on non-fasting days.

Solution: Fix this problem by making a meal plan specifically for your non-fasting days. Make sure the program balances each meal to contain 300 to 500 calories. This way, don't rely on guesswork to determine if you meet the requirements or not. Also, you won't have to skimp on calories for yourself.

Wrong Eating Window

There are different approaches to take toward intermittent fasting. You cannot try all these methods, so you have to choose one consistent with your lifestyle and weight loss goals. If you choose one that does not suit your lifestyle, you might see no fasting results.

For instance, if you typically hit the gym during weekdays or work overtime, the 5:2 diet may be too restrictive for you. At the end of each fasting window, you may end up feeling famished. This is a sure recipe for failure.

Solution: Choose an eating window that falls within the time you do the most strenuous activities in your life. If a 12-hour window is all you can do without triggering significant discomfort feelings, go ahead with it. Don't force yourself to do more than you can handle. You may also start with a 16-hour fast. The steps in the preceding chapter breaks down 16:8 fasting into small steps that make things easy for beginners.

Wrong Food Intake

Just because IF focuses on your mealtime instead of tracking macronutrients does not give you the room to fill your diet up with junk. You must still eat healthy while you are fasting. Eating the wrong food can obstruct your weight loss.

The wrong foods don't give you the nutrients your body needs to sustain itself. Nourishing your body with nutrient-rich whole foods is a must. The body finds those easier to break down during a fasting window, which improves satiation.

Do not use IF as an excuse to consume processed foods and sugar because they are not suitable for your body when it is in a fasted state.

Solution: Fill up your diet with healthy fats, complex carbs, lean protein, and more fiber. Refer back to chapters where the kind of healthy foods to eat during intermittent fasting has been explained. On the side, you can still consume some of your favorite less-healthy foods like ice cream and pizza, but make sure you do this in moderation.

Short Fasting Window

You are unlikely to get any results from an intermittent fasting plan if your fasting window is less than 12 hours a day. Shortening your daily eating window by 1 to 2 hours will make no difference. A short fasting window makes your body unable to complete all the phases in the fed-fast cycle. You need to change much of your regular eating routine.

Solution: To achieve success, you need to have at least a 12-hour fasting window. Most experts recommend a 14-hour window for women because it can be successful for most intermittent dieters. This does not mean you can't start with a longer eating window, but make sure it doesn't outweigh the fasting window. If anything, starting with a longer eating window means you can eventually work your way down as you get more familiar with intermittent fasting.

Meal-Skipping During Eating Window

You cannot skip meals during your eating window because that will cause extreme hunger during the fasting periods. That makes you more likely to break your fast. It is best to avoid this. Do not restrict yourself too much during any eating window. Otherwise, you may end up binge-eating the next fasting window. The result of this is too much caloric intake.

Solution: Eat until you are full during your eating windows, but don't overstuff yourself. Just make sure that you are satisfied. Also consider doing meal preps for the weekdays on weekends. By doing that, you are unlikely to skip meals even when you get busy or throw off your daily schedule.

Intense Workout

Often, many people mistake starting their intermittent fasting plan around the same time they just jump onto a new exercise regimen. Some boost their current plan because they believe that will help increase the rate at which they lose fat. Things do not work like that.

An intense workout while you are reducing your food intake is not ideal. Over-exercising while fasting causes your energy levels to drop as your hunger levels rapidly increase. You may consume more calories than you can expend during your eating window. Even with the intense exercise plan, don't be surprised if you get no noticeable changes.

Solution: Keep exercise light during fasting periods. If you are on the 5:2 plan, don't exercise during your fasting days. In general, make sure that you follow a challenging workout program, but make it enjoyable. If you feel ravenous on the days you exercise, it may mean you are overworking.

Insufficient Hydration

The importance of drinking enough water on fasting days cannot be overstated. Not getting enough fluid intake while you are on a fast can leave you feeling dehydrated. By not drinking sufficient water, you also miss out on the amazing benefits of water regarding satiating or suppressing hunger.

Solution: Drink 2 to 3 liters of water daily during fasting and non-fasting windows. And the best thing is that you can add some flavor to your fluid intake. Hot tea, iced tea, black coffee tea, stevia coffee, and seltzer water are some drinks that are approved for intermittent fasting. These drinks are non-caloric, meaning they won't add to your calorie intake no matter how much you drink them in a day.

Deviating From the Plan

Following an IF plan may be difficult for beginners who are not familiar with prolonged periods without eating anything. If you keep cheating on your plan or cutting corners because of hunger, it won't yield your expected results. It is much better to reevaluate yourself and your lifestyle to determine if time-restricted eating is for you or not.

Solution: Choose an IF plan that matches your lifestyle perfectly. That increases the likelihood of you following the plan consistently - despite obstacles.

Those are the most common problems people face when they start intermittent fasting. Suppose you address these problems and apply the solutions offered for each. In that case, you will start seeing noticeable changes in your body with your intermittent fasting plan.

As you continue fasting, you will learn some lessons that will change your perception about intermittent fasting and help build you into a better dieter and faster. What are these lessons?

The first lesson you might learn is that mindset is single-handedly your biggest obstacle. This dieting plan is simple and straightforward. Many people agree that it is one of the most straightforward dieting strategies to follow. All you have to do is *not eat until you wake up, eat once you get to work, eat again during lunch hours, and go about your business until dinner arrives again.*

But there is a mental barrier most people face when they attempt fasting. "Will it affect my thinking if I don't eat?" "If I don't eat, will I faint or fall sick?" "What will it be like? Can I do this?" These are some thoughts that run to and from your mind when you get started.

If you get past this mental barrier and questions, you will realize that nothing happens. Life will continue as before. You may not even feel like someone who has just made a huge lifestyle change. The only apparent difference will be the extra pounds falling off your body each week as your fasting progresses.

The things you have convinced yourself about, such as the hours you should eat or snack are perceptions. They don't matter in context. You eat breakfast at 7 a.m. because you were told to, not because you actually have to.

Forget what you think you know and readjust your mental space to accommodate your new lifestyle. The ability to think and act differently is the foundation to success in anything you try.

A second lesson you should expect to learn is that weight loss is easy. That is right – because eating less frequently means eating less overall. Because of this, most people on this diet end up losing fat.

Intermittent fasting offers you a simple way of cutting down on your weight by cutting down on total caloric intake without making a drastic change to your diet. And this is why many dieters enjoy fasting.

Even if you follow a plan that lets you eat two large meals at lunch and dinner, you end up consuming fewer calories than you usually would if you had three regular meals with snacks between.

Yes, muscle loss happens as you get older, but you might just be surprised at the results you see when you start time-restricted eating. If you follow your plan as you should, you may build and maintain your muscle mass which means you are burning fat rather than muscle.

There are several other personal lessons you will learn as you progress with your journey. Incorporate these into your life as you work on making intermittent fasting an integral part of your daily routine. Remember that intermittent fasting is more than just a dieting technique – it is a lifestyle.

Chapter 9: Exercises for Women Over 50

Chapter 5 mentioned that strength training, stability training, aerobic training, and flexibility training are a must in a workout routine for women over 50. While intermittent fasting helps you lose weight, you can improve your body with exercise the older you get. In other words, the right exercise regimen can help you turn back the years on your whole appearance.

Several studies have shown that exercise slows down the physiological aging clock and helps older people stay young. And although cardiovascular activities like walking, biking, cycling, and jogging are great for your heart and lung health, strength training is the real deal that provides what your body needs in its fifties.

Strength training is the best exercise for you because it helps you stay younger and more vital and keeps you functioning optimally as your body ages. To remain vibrant and self-sufficient for many more years to come, the strength training exercise below is your key to achieving that.

Experts recommend strength-training for older women because, after 50, the crucial things shift from building big biceps or achieving flat abs to maintaining a strong, lean, and healthy body that is less susceptible to injury and diseases.

Strength-training workouts can help you build bone density, add muscle mass, shed body fat, and improve your cognitive health. They also reduce the risk of chronic illnesses. These reasons explain why strength-training is a big deal for older women.

Even if you do only 20 to 30 minutes of training per day, you can notice considerable changes in your overall appearance and mental health. It often helps to have a physically active group of friends to exercise with. Check out workout classes in your local area, or simply bring friends together.

If you can afford to talk to a fitness expert, then speak to one – even if it is just for a session. In a single session, they can teach the proper form and how to move your body appropriately when trying strength-training workouts.

Forearm Plank

This exercise targets your shoulders and abdominals.

> 1. Start by lying on the floor. Let your forearms spread flat while your elbows are placed directly under your shoulders.

> 2. Raise your body off the ground and engage your core as you do this. Ensure that your forearms stay on the floor and your entire body forms a straight line from head to feet. Keep your core engaged, and don't let your hips move out of position. They should neither dip nor rise.

> 3. Hold still for 3o seconds instead of doing reps. If you feel uncomfortable or your lower back hurts, places your knees on the ground.

Modified Push-Up

This workout targets your shoulders, core, and arms.

1. Start in a kneeling position on a workout mat. Place both hands below your shoulders with your knees behind your hips. That way, your back takes an angled and long-form.

2. Tuck your toes under, tighten your core and slightly bend your elbows. Then slowly lower your chest toward the ground.

3. Look straight at the front of your fingertips, so the neck stays long.

4. Press your chest back to the initial position. Repeat these steps a few times.

Stability Ball Chest Fly

This workout targets your chest, back, glutes, and abdominals.

1. Hold two dumbbells to your chest. Position your shoulder blades and head directly on top of the stability ball. Keep the rest of your body in a tabletop pose. Check to see that your feet are hip-distance apart.

2. Raise the pair of dumbbells together straight above your chest, with the palms facing each other.

3. Slowly lower your arms out to the sides while slightly bending your elbows until they are about chest level.

4. Tighten your chest and bring your hands together back to the top.

Basic Squat

The basic squat workout is targeted at the glutes, hamstrings, and quads.

1. Stand upright with your feet apart. Maintain a hip-distance between both while your hips, knees, and toes all face forward. Hold a pair of dumbbells in both hands to increase the difficulty.

2. Stretch your buttocks outward as you bend your knees. Do this as if you are trying to sit on a chair. Ensure your knees are behind your toes and shift the weight on your heels.

3. Rise back up and repeat the workout a couple of times.

Shoulder Overhead Press

This workout is targeted at your biceps, back, and shoulders.

1. Pull your feet hip-distance apart. Bring your elbows out to your sides as you create a goal post position. Keep your dumbbells at the side of your head and tighten your abdominal muscles.

2. Slowly press the dumbbells until your arms are up straight. Return to the initial position with slow control. You can try this workout on a chair or a stability ball with your feet wide apart.

These five strength-training exercises are some of the easiest to perform. Incorporate one or two into your day-to-day workout routine.

Aerobic training makes a lot of difference to your workout programs. They exercise the large muscles in your body, which benefits your cardiovascular system and weight. Get in 20 minutes of aerobic exercise each training session, at least three days a week. Ensure that you pass the "talk test" when training. The "talk test" means working out at a pace that simultaneously allows you to have a conversation.

Stretching exercises are equally as important as strength training and aerobic training. It is a good idea to stretch a few times every day. The American College of Sports Medicine recommends stretching your major muscle groups two to three times a week at 60 seconds per exercise.

The point of stretches is to help you stay flexible as you get older. This improves mobility. Daily stretches can help your hips and hamstrings remain flexible despite aging. If your posture is causing any form of problem, form a habit of stretching your muscle groups every day. Also, if you sit at a desk all day, stretching can help lower back pain.

Simple Back Stretch

This simple stretching exercise is also called the "Standing cat camel." It is an excellent work-related stretch that can be completed in four easy steps.

1. Stand with your feet apart and your knees slightly bent. Make sure the distance between your feet is shoulder-width

2. Lean slightly forward with your hands just above your knees

3. Round your back to close your chest and curve your shoulders forward

4. Arch your back to open your chest and roll your shoulders backward

5. Repeat steps 1-4 multiple times

If you work a job that keeps you in the same position most of the time, consider trying the 2 minutes breaks to reverse the posture every 60 to 120 minutes.

Static Cat-Camel

A static stretch is when you stretch a muscle group to the fullest and hold it for about 15 to 30 seconds instead of repetitions. There is no harm in doing static stretches as long as you don't overdo them by remaining static until your muscles start to hurt. Below is a static version of the standing cat camel.

1. Lace your fingers together and turn your palms outwards in front of you

2. Curve your back and shoulders forward and reach your arms as far as you can with your palms

3. Hold still for 10 to 20 seconds

4. Now, release your fingers from one another, and twist your wrists behind your back gently

5. Raise your arms as high as they can behind your back. Do that without freeing your wrists so your shoulders roll back as your chest opens

Whether you are trying the static or dynamic stretch, you should never feel pain. What you should feel at any point is a stretch. So, don't stretch yourself beyond the range of motion your body needs.

Besides the strength-training and flexibility training exercises, you can try other workouts like the ones below.

Aerobic Interval Training

Aerobic interval training involves alternating between modern-to-high-intensity workouts with a recovery interval and a work interval. Your work interval is typically below 85 percent of the maximum heart rate. The recovery interval should bring your heart rate down to 110 bpm as you rest.

You can try this interval training with any aerobic activity of your choice, such as walking, running, jogging, or cycling. You can do it for 10 to 60 minutes. If you are new to interval training, do it for 10 minutes with a 2-minute recovery period.

Below is an AIT workout to try:

1. Warm-up your body for up to 10 minutes comfortably

2. Pick up speed or exertion to recovery level for 3 minutes

3. Increase speed for 1 to 2 minutes to increase your heart rate, but be careful not to exceed the 85% maximum heart rate

4. Return to recovery speed for 2 to 5 minutes

5. Repeat the work and recovery intervals during your chosen training length

You can try AITs two or more times each week.

Bicycle Crunch

The bicycle crunch is a classic exercise that works all of your core muscles at once, particularly the obliques and rectus abdominus. Try this exercise by following the steps below.

1. Lay flat on the floor and press your lower back to the ground

2. Place your hands behind your head gently without yanking your neck

3. Raise one of your knees to a 45-degree angle and let the other remain straight

4. Shift your legs back and forth as you would if you were cycling. Alternatively, extend one knee as you lift the other.

5. Touch your left elbow to your right knee and right elbow to left knee each time

6. Complete at least 20 to 50 reps on both sides. Be deliberate with your movements and remain steady.

7. Rest and complete two more sets before you wrap up

As you get stronger, up the number of reps you complete per set.

The Bridge

The bridge exercise targets your lower back, hamstrings, and gluteus muscles (buttocks). It can help improve spine stability and abdominal strength.

1. To assume the position, lie flat on your back and bend your knees. Keep your feet balanced and position your arms by your sides.

2. Inhale slowly and tighten your core and glutes while you lift your hips to form a straight line between your knees and shoulders.

3. Remain in the position for 15 to 60 seconds without dropping your lower back or buttocks.

4. If you feel like increasing this exercise's intensity, lift your leg as high as possible and hold still for 10 seconds.

As you become better at this exercise with practice, start increasing the duration of the pose.

Every bit of movement counts when you are in your 50s. If you find yourself too busy to commit to a standard workout program, find other ways to increase motion. All the extra steps you take add up to significant weight loss and overall health benefits.

Here are some ideas you can adopt to be in motion always:

- Take a dog for daily walks.

- Abandon the elevator and start using the stairs. Don't shout at people from the stairs - seize that opportunity to go on up.

- Get up whenever you have to talk with co-workers. Don't send texts or emails. Try walking to meetings regularly.

- Make brisk walking a habit - do it whenever you can. Always take comfortable shoes with you. That way, your feet can serve as your primary mode of transit.

Find a game, sport, or activity that requires mild to intense physical activity levels and make it your newest hobby. It is easy to commit to workout regimens when doing things you consider enjoyable.

Chapter 10: Recipes for Intermittent Fasting

Whether your eating window is within a 12-hour, 8-hour, or 4-hour range, you need to consume whole foods with powerful nutrients that can keep you feeling full and satisfied throughout your fasting window. The best approach is to try low-carb-high-protein recipes sure to make you feel nourished.

Naturally, you have to try different recipes for breakfast, lunch, and dinner. So, one by one, here are recipes ideal for different phases of your eating window.

Egg Scramble and Sweet Potatoes

Total cooking time: 25 minutes

Servings: 1

Ingredients:

- 1 sweet potato, diced
- Half cup of chopped onions
- Salt

- Pepper

- 2 tsp chopped rosemary

- 4 big eggs

- 2 spoons chopped chive

Directions:

1. Preheat your oven to 425 degrees Fahrenheit. Toss the diced potato, chopped onion, rosemary, salt, and pepper on a baking sheet. Apply cooking spray and allow to roast until soft and tender, for about 20 minutes.

2. Meanwhile, whisk the eggs and egg whites in a medium-sized bowl. Add a pinch of salt and pepper. Spritz with cooking oil and scramble the eggs in 5 minutes.

3. Sprinkle chopped chives and eat with the spuds.

One serving has 580 calories, 52g carbs, 44g protein, 9g fiber, and 20g fat.

PB & J Overnight Oats

Total time: 5 minutes (plus 8 hours for refrigeration)

Servings: 1

Ingredients:

- ¼ cup of fast-cooking rolled oats
- ½ cup of 2% milk
- ¼ cup of mashed raspberries
- 3 tablespoons of creamy peanut butter

Directions:

1. Add the oats, milk, mashed raspberries, and peanut butter together in a fairly-sized bowl. Stir gently until silky smooth.

2. Cover and put inside the refrigerator overnight. The next day, uncover and use whole raspberries as toppings.

One serving contains 455 calories, 36g carbs, 20g protein, 9g fiber, and 28g fat.

Turkish Egg Breakfast

Total time: 13 minutes

Servings: 2

Ingredients:

- 2 tablespoons olive oil
- ¾ cup of red bell pepper, diced
- ¾ cup eggplant, diced
- Pinch of salt and pepper
- 5 large eggs
- ¼ teaspoon paprika
- 1 whole-wheat pita
- 2 dollops plain yogurt
- Chopped cilantro

Directions:

1. Put a large nonstick skillet on moderate-high heat. Heat the olive oil. Add in the eggplant, bell pepper, salt, and pepper. Sauté until tender for about 7 minutes.

2. Lightly beat the eggs. Then, stir in the eggs and paprika. Add a little more salt and pepper to taste. Allow to cook and regularly stir until the eggs are scrambled.

3. Sprinkle the chopped cilantro and serve with one dollop of yogurt and pita.

One serving contains 470 calories, 26g carbs, 25g protein, 4g fiber, and 29g fat.

Almond Apple Spice Muffins

Total time: 15 minutes

Servings: 5

Ingredients:

- ½ stick butter
- 4 scoops of vanilla protein powder
- 2 cups of almond meal
- 4 eggs
- 1 cup of unsweetened applesauce
- 1 teaspoon allspice
- 1 tablespoon cinnamon
- 1 teaspoon cloves
- 2 tablespoons baking powder

Directions:

1. Preheat oven to 350 degrees. Using a small microwave-fitting bowl, melt the stick butter on low heat for about 30 seconds.

2. Thoroughly mix the remaining ingredients with the melted butter in a relatively large bowl—spritz two muffin tins with the cooking spray. If you have cupcake liners, use those.

3. Pour the mixture into muffin tins without overfilling. You should get ten muffins.

4. Put a tray in the oven and bake for 10 to 12 minutes. Do not overbake as this can make the muffins go too dry. Once baked, eject the tray from the oven. Put in the second tray and let the rest of the muffins bake the same way.

One serving contains 485 calories, 16g carbs, 40g protein: 5 g fiber, and 31g fat.

Greek Chickpea Waffles

Total time: 30 minutes

Servings: 2

Ingredients:

- ¾ cup of chickpea flour
- ½ teaspoon salt
- ½ teaspoon baking soda
- ¾ cup plain Greek yogurt (2%)
- 6 eggs
- Salt and pepper
- Tomatoes, olive oil, cucumbers, parsley, scallion, yogurt, lemon juice for serving (optional)

Directions:

1. Preheat oven to 200 degrees. Get a rimmed baking sheet and place a wire rack over to – put in the oven, heat one waffle irons per directions.

2. Beat together the flour, soda, and salt in a large bowl. In a different small bowl, beat together the egg and Greek yogurt. Mix the wet ingredients into the dry ones.

3. Softly cover the iron waffle with cooking spray, preferably a nonstick one. In groups, drop ¼ cup batter into each iron waffle section and cook until it turns to a golden-brown color. This will take around 4 to 5 minutes. Move the waffles to the oven to warm. Repeat with the rest of the batter.

4. Serve your waffles with a delicious tomato dressing or a simple mix of nut butter and berries.

One serving contains 415 calories, 24g carbs, 35g protein, 4g fiber, and 18g fat.

Turmeric Tofu Scramble

Total time: 15 minutes

Servings: 1

Ingredients:

- 1 portobello mushroom
- 3 cherry tomatoes
- 1 tablespoon olive oil
- 14-oz firm tofu
- Salt and pepper
- ¼ teaspoon ground turmeric
- A pinch of garlic powder
- ½ avocado, sliced thinly

Directions:

1. Preheat oven to 400 degrees. Place the mushroom and tomatoes on a baking sheet. Brush with olive oil. Add salt and pepper to season. Allow to roast until soft and tender – 10 minutes should do.

2. Additionally, add the tofu, garlic powder, turmeric, and a pinch of salt together in a moderately-sized bowl. Mash together with a fork.

3. Add 1 tablespoon olive oil to a large skillet. Pour in the mashed tofu mixture and let it cook. Stir until it takes a firm and egg-like form. This should be around 3 minutes.

4. Dish the tofu and serve with the roasted mushroom, tomatoes, and, if you like, avocado.

One serving contains 430 calories, 17g carbs, 21g protein, 8g fiber, and 33g fat.

Avocado Ricotta Power Toast

Total time: 5 minutes

Servings: 1

Ingredients:

- 1 whole-grain bread, sliced
- ¼ smashed avocado
- Pinch of crushed red pepper flakes
- 2 tablespoon ricotta
- Pinch flaky sea salt

Directions:

1. Toast the bread

2. Add avocado, crushed pepper flakes, ricotta, and sea salt as toppings

3. Serve with scrambled eggs, with a serving of fruit or yogurt

One serving contains 290 calories, 29g carbs, 10g protein, 10g fiber, and 17fg fat.

Apple and Cheddar Plus Mixed Greens

Total time: 5 minutes

Servings: 1

Ingredients:

- 2 tablespoon olive oil
- ¾ cup balsamic vinegar
- ¾ teaspoon ground black pepper
- ¼ teaspoon onion powder
- ¾ teaspoon garlic powder
- A pinch of salt
- 1 cup apple and cheddar
- 1 medium banana
- 2 cups mixed greens
- 1 tablespoon peanut butter

Directions

1. Mix the first five ingredients together in a medium-sized jar. Close the jar and shake it vibrantly until all the ingredients have mixed together well. Put in the refrigerator until it is lunchtime.

2. Chop the apple and cheddar cheese into cubes. Add the mixed greens together in a mixing bowl. Toss to mix together

3. Serve salad with a drizzle of vinaigrette

One serving contains 630 calories, 50g carbs, 10g protein, 6g fiber, and 47g fat.

Turkey Tacos

Total time: 25 minutes

Servings: 4

Ingredients:

- 2 teaspoons oil
- 1 finely chopped clove garlic
- 1 chopped red onion, small
- 1 tablespoon sodium-free taco seasoning
- 1 lb. lean turkey, ground
- 8 warmed whole-grain corn tortillas
- 1 sliced avocado
- ¼ cup of sour cream
- ½ cup Mexican cheese, shredded
- 1 cup lettuce, chopped
- Salsa, for serving

Directions:

1. Put a large skillet on medium-high to heat the oil. Pour in the onion and stir for 5 minutes until tender. Add the garlic and let it cook for 1 minute.

2. Pour in the turkey and allow to cook. Break up with a spoon at intervals until it is nearly brown, for about 5 minutes. Add a cup of water, plus the taco seasoning. Allow simmering until the water is reduced by more than half. This should take 7 minutes.

3. Fill up the corn tortillas with the turkey and use the sour cream, salsa, avocado, lettuce, and cheese as toppings.

One serving contains 470 calories, 30g carbs, 28g protein, 6g fiber, and 27g fat.

Chicken with Fried Cauliflower Rice

Total time: 35 minutes

Servings: 4

Ingredients:

- 2 tablespoon grapeseed oil
- 1 lb. pounded boneless, skinless chicken breast
- Eggs, beaten
- 2 finely chopped red bell peppers
- 1 finely chopped onion
- 2 carrots, finely chopped
- 2 finely chopped cloves of garlic
- 4 finely-chopped scallions, plus more for serving
- 4 cups of cauliflower rice
- ½ cup of thawed frozen peas
- 2 teaspoons of soy sauce, low sodium
- 2 teaspoons of rice vinegar
- Kosher salt and pepper, for taste

Directions:

1. Use a large, deep skillet that is over moderate-high. Heat the oil. Add the chicken breast and cook until it turns golden brown. This should take 3 or 4 minutes for both sides. Move chicken to a cutting board and allow to cool for 6 minutes before slicing. Add 1 tablespoon oil to the skillet. Pour in the eggs and aim for scrambled until you get the right set. Move to a bowl.

2. In the skillet, add the carrot, onion, and bell pepper and cook. Stir frequently until softened. Mix in the garlic and let it cook for 1 minute. Toss in the peas and scallions.

3. Add soy sauce, cauliflower, rice vinegar, salt, and pepper. Toss gently to mix all together. Allow the cauliflower "rice" to sit until it starts to brown. Do not stir.

4. Toss in the sliced chicken and scrambled eggs.

One serving contains 430 calories, 25g carbs, 45g protein, 7g fiber, and 16g fat.

Healthy Spaghetti Bolognese

Total time: 60 minutes

Servings: 4

Ingredients:

- 1 spaghetti squash, large
- ½ teaspoon garlic powder
- 2 tablespoon olive oil
- 1 finely chopped onion, small
- Kosher salt and pepper
- 1 ¼ lb. ground turkey
- 4 finely chopped cloves of garlic
- 3 cups of fresh tomato, diced
- 8 ounces of sliced cremini mushrooms
- 8 ounces of low-sodium, sugar-free tomato sauce
- Fresh basil, chopped

Directions:

1. Heat the oven to 400 degrees. Split the spaghetti squash in half and discard the seeds. Rub both halves with ½ teaspoon of oil each and add garlic powder and salt and pepper (1/4 tsp) to season. Put the skin side on a baking sheet (rimmed) and allows to cook until softened. This should take up to 4o minutes. After cooking, allow cooking for 10 minutes.

2. In the meantime, put a large skillet on moderate-high, and heat the remaining oil. Add the chopped onions and season with ¼ teaspoons of salt and pepper (each) and cook until softened for 6 minutes. Stir as it cooks.

3. Add turkey to the mix and break it up into smaller pieces as it cooks. Do this for about 7 minutes until browned. Put in the garlic, stir, and let it cook for 1 minute.

4. Gently push the mixture to one side and pour in the mushrooms on another side. Cook for 5 minutes until tender. Stir as it cooks. Mix together with the turkey. Pour in the tomatoes and tomato sauce. Leave it to simmer for 8 to 10 minutes.

5. Meanwhile, scoop out the spaghetti squash and serve on a plate. Scoop the turkey Bolognese over it and sprinkle the chopped basil if you wish.

One serving contains 45 calories, 31g carb, 32g protein, 6g fiber, and 23g fat.

Sheet Pan Steak

Total time: 50 minutes

Servings: 4

Ingredients:

- 1 lb. cremini mushrooms (small), trimmed and split into halves
- 1 ¼ lb. bunch broccolini, halved and trimmed
- 4 finely chopped cloves of garlic
- ¼ teaspoon of red pepper flakes
- 3 tablespoons of olive oil
- Kosher salt and pepper
- 1 ½ lb. New York strip steaks, trimmed
- 1 can low-sodium cannellini beans

Directions:

1. Preheat oven to 450 degrees. Using a large, rimmed baking sheet, toss the broccolini, mushrooms, oil, garlic, red pepper flakes, and salt and pepper. Put the sheet into the oven and allow to roast tenderly for 15 minutes.

2. Push the sheet containing the mushroom mixture to the edge to allow enough room for the steaks.

3. Add ¼ teaspoon of salt and pepper to the steaks to the season—place at the center of the pan. Roast the steaks until done to satisfaction. For medium-rare, roast for 7 minutes. Move the steaks to your cutting board and cool off for 5 minutes before you slice.

4. Rinse the beans and move them to the baking sheet. Toss to mix together. Allow roasting until thoroughly heated.

5. Serve the beans and vegetables with sliced steaks.

One serving is 465 calories, 26g carbs, 42g protein, 8g fiber, and 22g fat.

Wild Cajun Spiced Salmon

Total: 30 minutes

Servings: 4

Ingredients:

- 1 lb. Salmon Fillet, wild Alaskan
- ½ cauliflower head, cut into florets
- 1 broccoli head, cut into florets
- 3 tablespoons olive oil
- ½ teaspoon of garlic powder
- 4 tomatoes, medium and diced
- Sodium-free taco seasoning

Directions:

1. Preheat oven to 375 degrees. Put the salmon fillet in a reasonably large baking dish. Mix the taco seasoning with ½ cup of water in a smaller bowl. Add the mixture over the salmon and let it bake until thoroughly opaque. Do this for 12 to 15 minutes.

2. Meanwhile, use a food processor to pulse the broccoli and cauliflower until thoroughly chopped and "riced."

3. Put a large skillet on medium-high. Pour in the oil to heat. Put in the broccoli and cauliflower, then sprinkle the garlic powder. Toss and cook until softened. That should take 6 minutes.

4. Serve the salmon on the rice and add the tomatoes as toppings.

One serving contains 410 calories, 9g carbs, 42g protein, 3g fiber, and 23g fat.

Pork Chops with Bloody Mary Tomato Salad

Total time: 25 minutes

Servings: 4

Ingredients

- 2 tablespoons red wine vinegar
- 2 tablespoons olive oil
- 2 teaspoons dry-squeezed horseradish
- 2 teaspoons of Worcestershire sauce
- ½ teaspoon tabasco
- Kosher salt
- ½ teaspoon of celery seeds
- 1 pint of halved cherry tomatoes
- 2 thinly-sliced celery stalks
- ½ finely-sliced red onion, small
- Pepper
- 4 (2 ¼ lb.) small pork chops
- 1 little green-leaf lettuces, with torn leaves
- ¼ cup finely-chopped flat-leaf parsley

Directions:

1. Heat your grill to moderate-high. Using a large bowl, mix the oil, vinegar, horseradish, Worcestershire sauce, Tabasco, celery seeds, salt together. Toss the tomatoes, onion, and celery together.

2. Add ½ teaspoon salt and pepper to the pork chops to season. Grill for 5 to 7 minutes on each side until cooked and golden brown.

3. Fold the parsley inside the tomatoes and dish over the pork and greens.

4. Serve with potatoes or mashed cauliflower.

One serving contains 400 calories, 8g carbs, 39g protein, 3g fiber, and 23g fat.

Pork Tenderloin with Butternut Squash and Brussels Sprouts

Total time: 50 minutes

Servings: 4

Ingredients:

- 1 ¾ trimmed pork tenderloin
- Pepper
- Salt
- 2 sprigs thyme, fresh
- 3 tablespoon canola oil
- 2 peeled garlic cloves
- 4 cups butternut squash, diced
- 4 cups of halved and cut Brussels sprouts

Directions:

1. Preheat oven to 4oo degrees. Put the tenderloin in a large bowl and season all over with salt and pepper. Put a big iron cast pan on medium-high heat and pour in 1 tablespoon oil. Heat until it shimmers, then add in the tenderloin and stir until it turns golden brown on every side. This should take up to 12 minutes—dish into a plate.

2. Add the garlic, thyme, and remaining oil to the pan and cook until the aroma comes out for 1 minute. Pour in the Brussels sprouts, butternut squash, and a large pinch of salt and pepper. Cook and occasionally stir for about 6 minutes until the veggies are slightly browned.

3. Put the tenderloin over the vegetables and place everything inside the oven. Allow roasting until the veggies are tender and the tenderloin is thoroughly cooked. You

could insert a meat thermometer into the tenderloin to check the degree. It should be up to 140 degrees.

4. Put on oven mittens and take out the pan from the oven. Let the tenderloin cool off for 5 minutes before you slice and serve with the tender vegetables. Toss the greens with balsamic vinegar to serve as a side dish.

One serving contains 400 calories, 25g carbs, 44g protein, 6g fiber, and 15g fat.

Grilled Lemon Salmon

Total time: 27 minutes

Servings: 4

Ingredients:

- ½ teaspoon pepper
- 2 teaspoons fresh dill
- ½ teaspoon garlic powder
- ½ teaspoon salt
- ½ lbs. salmon fillets
- 1 chicken bouillon cube
- ¼ cup of brown sugar
- 3 tablespoons water
- 3 tablespoons oil
- 3 tablespoons soy sauce
- 4 finely chopped green onions
- 1 thinly-sliced lemon
- 2 ring-sliced onions

Directions:

1. Sprinkle the fresh dill, salt, pepper, and garlic powder over the salmon fillet.

2. Put inside a shallow glass pan

3. Add the chicken bouillon, soy sauce, sugar, and green onions together. Mix thoroughly.

4. Pour the mixture over the salmon fillet

5. Cover for 1 hour and allow to chill.

6. Drain the marinade

7. Place on preheated grill on medium heat with the lemon and oil over it.

8. Cover and allow to cook for 15 minutes or until the fish is done.

One serving contains 285 calories, 7.1 carbs, 20.3g protein, 0.5g fiber, and 19.8g fat.

Strawberry-Avocado Smoothie

Servings: 1

- 1 pound of strawberries, fresh or frozen
- 1 ½ cup of unsweetened almond milk
- 1 big, ripe avocado

Blend all the ingredients together until you achieve a smooth and refined taste.

One serving contains 190 calories, 28g carbs, 3g protein, 6g fiber, and 9g fat.

Creamy Chocolate Smoothie with MCT Oil

Servings: 1

- ½ cup of coconut full-fat coconut milk. You may substitute it with heavy whipping cream.

- ½ cup of peeled and seeded avocado

- ½ teaspoon of vanilla extract

- 2 tablespoons of cocoa powder

- Pinch of salt

- ½ cup of ice

- 1 tablespoon of MCT oil (or coconut oil)

- Non-caloric sweetener to taste

Blend all together, minus the ice, until smooth. If needed, add 2 tablespoons of water until you get the desired consistency. Add ice and blend until it becomes creamy.

One serving contains 595 calories, 19g carbs, 10g protein, 11g fiber, and 55g fat.

LCHF Green Protein Smoothie

Servings: 2

- 1 cup of fresh spinach leaves
- 1 ½ teaspoon of freshly-squeezed lemon juice
- ½ cup of peeled and seeded avocado
- 1 tablespoon of MCT oil
- 1 scoop of protein powder, low-carb
- 1 ½ teaspoon of flaxseed powder
- 1 teaspoon vanilla extract
- ¼ cup of water – adjustable as needed
- 5 ice cubes

Mix all the ingredients in the smoothie blender and blend until you get a smooth taste.

One serving contains 140 calories, 8.6g carbs, 4g protein, 3.8g fiber, and 10.8g fat.

Cinnamon Smoothie with Protein

Servings: 1

- 1 cup of unsweetened coconut or almond milk
- 1 scoop of protein powder, low-carb
- 1 tablespoon of MCT oil
- 4 ice cubes
- ½ teaspoon of cinnamon

Mix all ingredients together and blend till it is smooth. For a thicker and creamier consistency, replace ¼ cup of almond milk with ¼ heavy whipped cream.

Incorporate these tasty recipes into your intermittent fasting meal plan to ensure you don't consume too much or too few calories.

One serving contains 160 calories, 31g carbs, 5g protein, 4g fiber, and 3g fat.

Chapter 11: Balancing Intermittent Fasting and Your Social Life

Intermittent fasting can have a significant impact on your social life. You may not realize that a considerable aspect of your social life is built on meals and drinks. When you hang out with friends, you have a drink or two. When you have a meeting with coworkers at a restaurant, you eat to your heart's content.

Most of the social activities you engage in with the people in your life revolve around caloric intake. Naturally, this poses a challenge to your intermittent fasting journey. How do you navigate the intricacies of social life without affecting your resolution to meet your weight loss goals with extended fasting?

To maintain a balance between your social life and your weight loss journey, you have to follow only three rules. These rules are simple:

- Compromise
- Undertake
- Explain

The first is "compromise," which you may consider the act of making sacrifices to satisfy another person. It is an integral part of integrating IF perfectly into your social life. As crucial as compromise is, though, it should always come last. Do not resort to it until you have no other choice.

You cannot compromise your fasting every time you have a hangout with friends or family. Doing that all of the time is merely undermining the importance of your weight loss goals. It is akin to holding yourself back from success.

Understand when and when not to make compromises. But also, know that your IF lifestyle should not affect other aspects of your life adversely. Your social life shouldn't suffer because you are trying to lose extra weight. Your loved ones should also understand your journey and endeavor to make compromises of their own when necessary.

The second rule is "undertake." This essentially means taking over the execution of any planned, upcoming social events with family or friends. Doing this gives you more control over what you consume at such events. Also, you can use that opportunity to choose activities that cannot affect your fasting window.

Fortunately, intermittent fasting itself is a flexible diet, which means that you just need to tweak a little here and there whenever necessary. If you follow the 16:8 plan, that makes life even easier for you.

Finally, "explain" means you should outrightly tell friends and family whenever you are on a fast. Sometimes, explaining what you are doing is the key to getting them to accommodate your new lifestyle. You can even introduce interested loved ones to fasting. Having a group of people interested in the same thing can make a difference in your life as you become increasingly acclimatized to extended fasting.

Once you get them to understand why you are on that journey, they will do their best to support your progress. Don't be surprised when they start sending texts to let you know that your fasting window is still on and you "shouldn't eat that apple!"

And you can find people to fast with. Regardless of the approach you take to fasting, you can quickly get one or two people to fast together.

Conclusion

As you have learned throughout this book, weight loss via intermittent fasting is authentic and achievable. Being a woman in your 50s, losing weight need not be an arduous task. You can reap tons of benefits from fasting, and weight loss is just one of those benefits. Finding an approach suitable for you is as simple as ABC, thanks to the many intermittent fasting variations.

All you need to succeed in your intermittent fasting journey is to stick to everything you have learned in this book. Follow every rule, tip, and technique diligently, and you might just become the fittest 50-year-old lady you have ever come across. Good luck!

Here's another book by Daron McClain that you might like

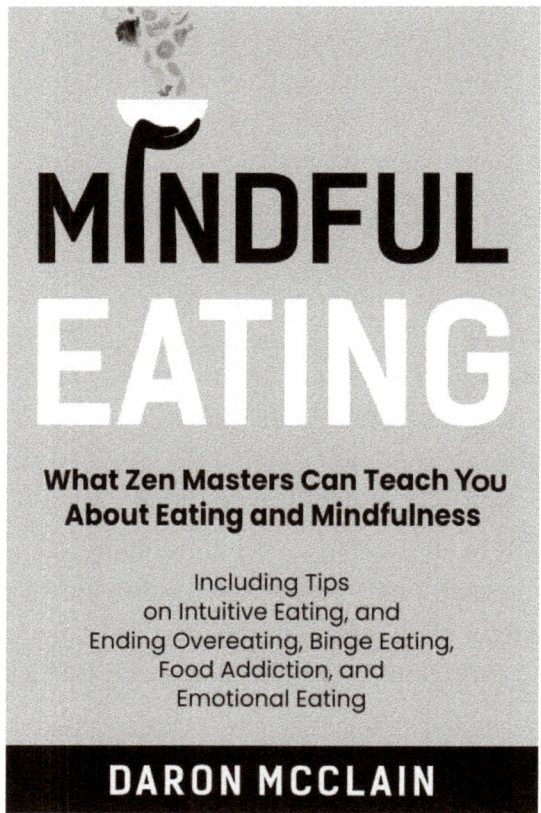

References

CenterForDiscoveryED. (2019, February 5). The Dangers of Intermittent Fasting - Center For Discovery. Center for Discovery. https://centerfordiscovery.com/blog/the-dangers-of-intermittent-fasting

Chuang, J.-C., & Zigman, J. M. (2010). Ghrelin's Roles in Stress, Mood, and Anxiety Regulation. *International Journal of Peptides, 2010*. https://www.hindawi.com/journals/ijpep/2010/460549/

Collier, R. (2013). Intermittent fasting: the science of going without. Canadian Medical Association Journal, 185(9), E363–E364. https://www.cmaj.ca/content/185/9/E363

Crane, M. M., Jeffery, R. W., & Sherwood, N. E. (2016). Exploring Gender Differences in a Randomized Trial of Weight Loss Maintenance. American Journal of Men's Health, 11(2), 369–375.

de Cabo, R., & Mattson, M. P. (2019). Effects of Intermittent Fasting on Health, Aging, and Disease. *New England Journal of Medicine, 381*(26), 2541–2551. https://www.nejm.org/doi/10.1056/NEJMra1905136

Research on intermittent fasting shows health benefits. (2020, February 27). National Institute on Aging. https://www.nia.nih.gov/news/research-intermittent-fasting-shows-health-benefits

Stockman, M.-C., Thomas, D., Burke, J., & Apovian, C. M. (2018). Intermittent Fasting: Is the Wait Worth the Weight? Current Obesity Reports, 7(2), 172–185. https://link.springer.com/article/10.1007/s13679-018-0308-9

Tello, M. (2018, June 26). Intermittent fasting: Surprising update - Harvard Health Blog. Harvard Health Blog.

https://www.health.harvard.edu/blog/intermittent-fasting-surprising-update-2018062914156

"Can You Boost Your Metabolism?" Mayo Clinic, 2017, www.mayoclinic.org/healthy-lifestyle/weight-loss/in-depth/metabolism/art-20046508.

"Healthline: Medical Information and Health Advice You Can Trust." Healthline.com, 2000, www.healthline.com/.

https://www.facebook.com/WebMD. "Do Men Lose Weight Faster than Women?" WebMD, WebMD, 13 Oct. 2015, www.webmd.com/diet/features/do-men-lose-weight-faster-than-women#1.

NCBI. "National Center for Biotechnology Information." Nih.gov, 2019, www.ncbi.nlm.nih.gov/.

PubMed Labs. "PubMed Labs." PubMed Labs, 2019, pubmed.ncbi.nlm.nih.gov/.

Shiffer, Emily. "12 Reasons You're Not Losing Weight While Doing Intermittent Fasting, according to an RD." Women's Health, 24 Mar. 2020, www.womenshealthmag.com/weight-loss/a31816703/not-losing-weight-intermittent-fasting/.